URBAN PLANNING & PUBLIC HEALTH
A CRITICAL PARTNERSHIP

URBAN PLANNING & PUBLIC HEALTH
A CRITICAL PARTNERSHIP

MICHAEL R. GREENBERG, PhD
DONA SCHNEIDER, PhD, MPH

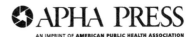
APHA PRESS
AN IMPRINT OF AMERICAN PUBLIC HEALTH ASSOCIATION

American Public Health Association
800 I Street, NW
Washington, DC 20001-3710
www.apha.org

Georges C. Benjamin, MD, FACP, FACEP (Emeritus), Executive Director

Printed and bound in the United States of America
Book Production Editor: Maya Ribault
Typesetting: The Charlesworth Group
Cover Design: Abduallahi Abdulgader
Printing and Binding: Sheridan Books

Library of Congress Cataloging-in-Publication Data

Names: Greenberg, Michael R., author. | Schneider, Dona, 1946- author. |
    American Public Health Association, issuing body.
Title: Urban planning and public health : a critical partnership / by Michael
    R. Greenberg, Dona Schneider.
Description: Washington, DC : American Public Health Association, [2017] |
    Includes bibliographical references and index.
Identifiers: LCCN 2017041932 (print) | LCCN 2017042215 (ebook) | ISBN
    9780875532905 (e-book) | ISBN 9780875532899 (pbk.)
Subjects: | MESH: Urban Health | City Planning | Public Health | Public
    Policy | Environment Design | Safety | United States
Classification: LCC RA566.7 (ebook) | LCC RA566.7 (print) | NLM WA 380 | DDC
    362.1/042–dc23
LC record available at https://lccn.loc.gov/2017041932

Dedicated to our grandchildren—Layla and Lola Suggs; Amelia, Max, and Zane Wilkerson; Faith Pappas; Eli and Willie Jacob-Perez; and Anna, Lily, Maggie, and Matthew Schneider—along with the millions of other children who will benefit from the ties between urban planning and public health practice being strengthened and tightened.

TABLE OF CONTENTS

FOREWORD

While completing my higher education, I had the opportunity to attend a university that had strong programs in engineering, architecture, design, the biological sciences, and applied technology. Consequently, I spent a lot of time with a range of people who thought about how to build things and what the human impact of building would be. In fact, my college roommate was an urban planner. I became a physician and eventually entered public health practice. Throughout that time, I watched my friend develop his skills as a planner, and we shared many conversations about the health implications of his fascinating work. Looking back on these discussions and where our life experiences have taken us, I see with striking clarity the intersection of our respective fields: public health and urban planning. I did not appreciate the commonality of our goals during those first years in college. But today I understand that while we were both on different career paths, at the end of the trail was a shared responsibility to build healthy communities.

The phrase "building healthy communities" is more than a symbolic one. It actually means ensuring the physical and environmental aspects of where we live, work, and play: we select safe locations, we build to protect, and we design to promote wellness. These three core aspects of the built environment define the intersection of urban planning and public health. While each professional sees a new development project through the lens of his or her own respective field, there is a commonality of purpose that can be achieved if both approach the project from a healthy community frame, beyond the usual considerations of development or regulatory responsibility.

One of the biggest challenges for both urban planners and public health practitioners is optimizing the advantage of having the combined experience of both disciplines at the table when designing and developing a truly health-driven project. A lot of what we do is experience-driven, and while taught in both schools of public health and urban planning, many of the people that practice public health and urban planning come from a variety of related disciplines and may not have received formal training in public health or urban planning.

This book is written to give both public health practitioners and urban planners a common understanding of this critical partnership and what they can achieve by working together. It offers context by describing the historic roots of both professions, provides an overview of the most important tools used in decision-making, and employs case studies to reinforce the essential common approach of safety, health protection, and health promotion. This book is indispensable reading for everyone charged with building healthy communities.

Georges C. Benjamin, MD
Executive Director
American Public Health Association

PREFACE

We have collectively engaged in research projects that weave together public health and planning principles, practice, data, and tools in order to inform practice for more than 75 years. We have also taught and built curricula in a school that offers planning, public health, and policy degrees. When the American Public Health Association (APHA) approached us in a conversation about writing this book we were intrigued. An advantage of our multidisciplinary experience is that we have the ability to cover a broad range of subjects; unfortunately this is also a disadvantage because books need a focus.

After much consultation and deliberation among the authors, reviewers, and APHA in-house experts, we made several decisions. The main audiences for this book are practitioners in public health and planning, and students who are likely to become practitioners in the near future. We agreed to focus on typical events that require cross-collaborations of planning and public health professionals such as the following scenario:

> You are a public health and/or planning practitioner working in a government agency, not-for-profit, or company. A colleague comes into your office, probably the director of the organization, and says: "The Friendly Development Company has approached us with a proposal to build 150 townhomes for seniors on the old Jones & Jones roofing shingles plant adjacent to the Smithtown River. The site, as you know, has been abandoned and fenced in for more than 20 years. What should we do?"

Practitioners charged with answering this type of question have to know (1) what to do and (2) how to do it. If they are not familiar with the intersection of land-use planning and/or environmental health, they need to get up to speed on the latest analytical ideas, data, and tools. In the hypothetical case above, they need to know

- The history of the site
- If it is contaminated
- Legal status of the site
- Whether there are engineered structures on the site that could be compromised
- The risk associated with building a facility for seniors on this property
- The likelihood of the site flooding
- The extent of nearby shopping, medical facilities, and transit
- The answers to many other important questions that are discussed elsewhere in the book

We understood when we undertook this project that our readers would be unlikely to have advanced quantitative or qualitative analysis skills. They would also want examples at different geographic scales (local, regional, and national) and a carefully selected webliography that would allow them to access additional relevant data, tools, and examples.

We did not want to provide an exhaustive history of the professions and how they worked together. However, we also knew that our readers were likely to be familiar with the history of their own field but not of the other. Thus, Part I offers three chapters that include some history, but the focus is to set the context for how professionals in each field think and work—important information for understanding the tools and case studies that follow in Part II.

In Part II, the case studies provided are real, not hypothetical ones designed to highlight a select set of tools. In other words, we believe we have avoided the problem of the tail (the tools) wagging the dog (the case study). Because the cases are real, the tools described are employed in the context of the cases. This also means the tools have real limitations that we have been careful to point out. This approach, we believe, will prevent the confusion of trying to fit problems to the tool (the "get a bigger hammer" approach) rather than selecting the appropriate tools to address the problem.

If we have been successful, readers will keep this book on their shelf and refer to it as new challenges emerge. The 18 tool sets are applicable to a wide range of challenges. While the case studies will eventually age, they should be handy and interesting references for readers.

Michael R. Greenberg, PhD
Dona Schneider, PhD, MPH

ACKNOWLEDGMENTS

We could not have imagined writing this book two decades ago. With rare exceptions, the relationship between urban planning and public health was not a priority for either field. In some cases there was resistance to even talking about it at either faculty meetings or professional conferences. For example, in the early 1990s we wrote an article about the need to retie the knot between the disciplines. It was rejected by both a public health and a planning journal before eventually being published as a history piece.

Later that decade, as new environmental health issues were identified and older ones were not entirely resolved, books and articles began to call for re-engaging planning and public health in a serious relationship. We specifically acknowledge three brilliantly written books for motivating many practitioners and professors of both disciplines to make retying the knot a priority:

- *Toward the Healthy City* by Jason Coburn (Cambridge, MA: MIT Press; 2009)
- *Urban Sprawl and Public Health: Designing, Planning, and Building for Healthy Communities* by Howard Frumkin, Lawrence Frank, and Richard Jackson (Washington, DC: Island Press; 2004)
- *The Geography of Nowhere: The Rise and Decline of America's Man-Made Landscape* by James Kunstler (New York, NY: Touchstone; 1995)

At the same time, some key organizations stepped up to make re-engaging the professions a priority, most specifically the following:

- American Public Health Association (APHA)
- American Planning Association (APA)
- Centers for Disease Control and Prevention (CDC)
- Congress for the New Urbanism (CNU)
- National Association of County and City Health Officials (NACCHO)
- U.S. Environmental Protection Agency (EPA)
- World Health Organization (WHO)

We acknowledge the special contributions made by the above individuals and organizations, and we call for ongoing efforts to build an even larger network of intersecting practices to make healthy cities, communities, and environments for us all.

I. UNDERSTANDING THE PROFESSIONS

A CRITICAL PARTNERSHIP

The growing partnership between public health and urban planning in the early 21st century renews a critical relationship born out of the human health and environmental distresses of the Industrial Revolution. We begin with limited but essential context about the growth and impacts of urbanization and industrialization, focusing on infectious diseases, fire, housing, fresh water, and sanitation. We then describe the growth of the fields of planning and public health as distinct disciplines, their separation and their recent reconnection.

The Rise of Urban America

The Industrial Revolution brought with it jobs and economic growth, but it also brought skies filled with smoke, contaminated water supplies, wretched housing conditions, and the multiple diseases associated with crowding. The promise of jobs drew waves of immigrants who would dig canals, lay railroad tracks, and staff the industrial plants that fueled the engines of commerce. The urban poor slept in shifts in basements and boarding houses, shoveled out the mounds of night soil that accumulated between housing structures, and did what they could to survive. Average life expectancy for whites in the United States during the mid-1800s was only 40 years of age, but that was fully a decade longer than only half a century before. Unfortunately, the average life expectancy for American blacks, many of whom were enslaved, was only 23 years.[1]

Before 1832, the diseases that took the most American lives within the shortest period of time were epidemics of smallpox, measles, and yellow fever. Smallpox and measles are uniquely human contagions and these were understood, even in early times, to be spread from an infected individual to others who were susceptible. Yellow fever, however, is an acute, vector-borne viral illness carried by mosquitos that breed in standing water. The disease was widely feared because it seemed to arise spontaneously with no known cause, often leading to liver involvement and jaundice, which turned skin yellow. Widespread fear of yellow fever was justified as the disease killed 5,000 persons in Philadelphia, Pennsylvania, in 1793, with additional large-scale epidemics in the ensuing years in the port cities of New York, New York; Boston, Massachusetts; Baltimore, Maryland; Norfolk, Virginia; and New Orleans, Louisiana. The disease then spread up the Mississippi River Valley where yellow fever caused more than 20,000 deaths in the summer of 1878 alone.

Other infectious diseases plaguing many Americans of the time included another vector-borne disease, malaria, and typhoid fever, a bacterial infection caused by *Salmonella typhi*. These diseases always weakened and sometimes killed their victims, but they arose as smaller outbreaks and created less panic among the populace. They created concern, however, as they did not only strike the poor. For example, seven American presidents are documented as having contracted malaria (George Washington, James Monroe, Andrew Jackson, Zachary Taylor, Abraham Lincoln, Ulysses S. Grant, and James A. Garfield) and most suffered from recurrent bouts of the disease throughout their lives. President William H. Harrison died of typhoid fever at age 68 after serving only one month in the White House. A second U.S. president, Zachary Taylor, also died while in office of a disease that some believe may have been typhoid.[2]

In 1832, cholera reached the United States for the first time, killing 3,515 persons in New York City within months. The disease then reached into the port cities of the East Coast, through the nation's new canal systems, up the Hudson Valley, into the Great Lakes, and up the Mississippi River Valley.[3] Cholera is an acute diarrheal disease that can kill within hours, yet is it totally preventable by providing populations with clean water and protecting them from exposure to sewage contaminated with *Vibrio cholerae*. Unfortunately, the nation was not yet ready to provide such services to its citizens. As medical geographer Gerald Pyle noted in his book describing how cholera spread throughout the early United States:

> In 1832, the United States was barely more than a frontier country. Most major cities of the time were periodically drowned in mud. Pigs roamed the streets of New York. Sanitation as it is now known was virtually unheard of.[3]

The new nation did not remain a frontier country for long, and it was quickly becoming clear that epidemics were a major threat to urban development. Early theories of disease linked the outbreaks with both contagion and the "filth factor" associated with poor living conditions. Thus, efforts to deal with epidemics focused on quarantine. New York City opened a quarantine station on Bedloe's Island in 1738; Philadelphia opened one 10 miles south of the city in 1793 (see Figure 1.1).[5] By the end of that century, all of the port cities along the Atlantic coast had quarantine laws to prevent those with or exposed to disease from entering American cities.

Another prevailing theory of disease of the time was that miasma ("bad air") caused sporadic outbreaks. Supporters of the miasma theory assumed that emanations from filth were inherent in urban areas (particularly from rotting garbage, dead animals, offal, and sewage) and that addressing these issues would prevent future outbreaks. The answer for some—particularly physicians and social activists—was the Sanitary Reform Movement.

A cogent argument for sanitary reform was put forth in Lemuel Shattuck's *Report of the Sanitary Commission of Massachusetts* in 1850.[6] Although not universally accepted, Shattuck's arguments spurred the creation of state boards of health in Massachusetts (1869),

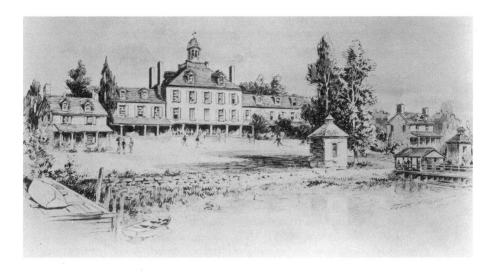

Source: Reprinted from the Library of Congress Prints and Photographs Division.[4]
Note: The site was placed on the National Register of Historic Places in 1972 and remains open to visitors today.

Figure 1.1. The [Philadelphia] Lazaretto, Drawn by Frank H. Taylor in 1895

California (1870), the District of Columbia (1871), Virginia (1872), Minnesota and Michigan (1873), Maryland (1874), and Alabama (1875).[7] Growing cities, however, maintained their own boards of health rather than waiting for state efforts to address their needs. City boards of health often advocated but were not always successful, in bringing clean water supplies to their inhabitants and removing human and animal wastes. Boards of health also supported paving major streets and providing sewers to remove runoff. They advocated improving crowded and dangerous housing conditions and encouraged clean milk stations to reduce infant mortality. Some of the early events that improved human health and safety, along with overall living conditions in U.S. cities, are listed in Table 1.1.

The United States expanded demographically, economically, and geographically over the 19th and early 20th centuries. Westward expansion turned prairie into farmland and timber into building materials for new towns and rail lines. Ample waterpower and coal fueled new industries and steam engines replaced slower water and overland transport. Immigration provided cheap labor and the number of smokestacks sprouting up in an area was seen as a sign of economic growth. By 1860 there were 392 urban places in the United States, with nine cities populated with more than 100,000 persons. By 1900 there were 1,737 urban places, with 38 cities populated with more than 100,000 persons. Indeed, New York City transformed from 45,000 inhabitants in 1800 to a metropolis of more than 4 million in 1900, with more than 250,000 persons transported by ferries across the Hudson River each day.[8]

Municipal water supplies attempted to keep pace with burgeoning demands, but sanitary conditions and potable water did not improve at the same rapid rate. The first

Table 1.1. Early Milestones for Public Health and Urban Planning in the United States

Year	Event
1802	Philadelphia, Pennsylvania, opens the first city-wide waterworks in the United States.
1803	The first gas lights appear on a street in Newport, Rhode Island.
1842	The Croton Aqueduct begins supplying water from Westchester County to New York City.
1854	New York Common Council rules that homes have to be connected to sewer lines. In 1857, two-thirds of New Yorkers still have backyard and basement privies that overflow.
1855	Chicago, Illinois, becomes the first city with a comprehensive sewer plan.
1857	Frederick Law Olmsted and Calvert Vaux win the design competition for New York City's Central Park, aimed at providing open space for city residents.
1863	The Association for the Improvement of the Condition of the Poor reports that 18,000 people in New York City live in cellar apartments with floors consisting of putrid mud.
1866	The New York State Legislature creates the Metropolitan Board of Health with authority to conduct house-to-house inspections, remove nuisances, and order cleanups.
1867	Chicago opens new waterworks valves, taking water from two miles out in Lake Michigan rather than the polluted Chicago River.
c. 1880	The first U.S. municipal smoke abatement laws are devised so that local boards of health could enforce them as nuisance statutes.
1880	The first electric streetlights are installed in Wabash, Indiana.
1881	Chicago becomes the first American city to create a local ordinance regulating smoke discharge. Cincinnati, Ohio; Pittsburgh, Pennsylvania; and St. Louis, Missouri, follow by 1893.
1881	New York City creates a Department of Street Cleaning.
1881	The American Water Works Association is founded to promote public health, safety, and welfare through the quality and quantity of water delivered to the public.
1890	Jacob Riis publishes *How the Other Half Lives*, eye-opening photojournalism that stimulates housing reform.
1891	The first successful indoor public bathing facility opens in New York City, a response to the concern that more than 90 percent of tenement residents had no baths.
1908	The first continuous chlorination of drinking water in the United States begins serving Jersey City, New Jersey.

American city to build waterworks to serve its population was Philadelphia in 1802. By 1860, the 16 largest cities in the nation all had waterworks, although water for drinking and food preparation was often contaminated and served as an efficient means for delivering water-borne pathogens, particularly typhoid and cholera. Water pressure was often insufficient for fighting fires, a significant threat for urban residents.[9]

Fire

Fires in 19th-century cities were common. As cities exploded in size, their populations crammed into close living quarters, usually with no building codes. Wooden structures with no indoor plumbing prevailed and access to water was usually restricted to a common tap. There were few fire hydrants and, where they did exist, hose connections and threaded couplings on the hydrants were not standardized. Municipalities had no interest in taxing residents to provide such public services and no firefighting unit wanted to abandon its own coupling system.

The Great Fire of New York City of 1845 spread for more than 10 hours, taking with it all wood-frame structures for 17 city blocks. It caused $20 million in property damage and the deaths of 30 people.[10] In 1871, the Great Chicago Fire raged for two days, leaving a four-mile path of destruction that included the entire business district. The result was $222 million in damages, fully one-third of the Windy City's total valuation. Losses included 73 miles of roads, 120 miles of sidewalk, 2,000 lampposts, and 17,500 buildings. About 300 people lost their lives and more than 100,000 were left homeless by the conflagration.[11]

Some of the major fire events in early U.S. cities are listed in Table 1.2. Not included in the table are losses to cities burned during military campaigns (e.g., Buffalo, New York; Atlanta, Georgia; and Washington, D.C.), by wildfires (e.g., Peshtigo, Wisconsin), or that may have taken many lives but were restricted to a single location (e.g., the Hoboken Docks Fire of 1900 or the Triangle Shirt Fire of 1911).

Great destruction makes for great opportunities for rebuilding and redesigning cities for safer and healthier conditions. The Great Fire of New York City of 1845 was fueled by gale-force winds. Freezing temperatures that day forced firefighters to chop through the ice on the East River to access water to fight the fire. Unfortunately, the water froze in the fire hoses. This lack of access to water spurred the city to create a new municipal water supply, the Croton Aqueduct. The city also implemented new building codes and firefighting practices.[11]

After the Great Chicago Fire of 1871, Frederick Law Olmsted reported on the causes in the *Nation*. He noted Chicago's weakness in trying to outbuild New York City. The result was wooden structures with thin walls and parapets simply for show, with flammable flat roofs covered with tarred felt and pebbles in order to support large advertising. Olmsted flatly stated that plain brick was better than wood for creating fire-resistant buildings.[12] Chicago city managers responded by passing building codes requiring the use of fireproof materials for new construction. Those who could not afford brick or stone rebuilt with terra cotta clay roofs to improve fire resistance. By the mid-1880s, Chicago was considered one of the most fireproof cities in the nation.[13]

The Great Fire of Boston in 1872 destroyed most of the city's downtown. The fire spread because the fireboxes had been locked to stop the rash of false alarms, sorely hindering firefighters' response. As in Chicago, the Great Fire of Boston jumped easily from building to building because the most common construction type was wood with a flammable flat roof. The city also lacked sufficient water to fight the fire as the hydrant couplings were not standardized and there was low water pressure in the city's old water pipes. City planners recommended that before rebuilding, the city should widen downtown streets, increase water mains in size, and increase the number of hydrants. One year

Table 1.2. Major Fire Events in U.S. Cities

Year	Event
1776	The First Great Fire of New York City destroys approximately one-third of the city.
1788	The First Great Fire of New Orleans, Louisiana, destroys 856 of the 1,100 structures in the city.
1794	The Second Great Fire of New Orleans destroys 212 structures in the French Quarter. New construction includes courtyards, brick walls, and iron balconies.
1805	The Great Fire of Detroit, Michigan, levels the city except for one stone fort. The city rebuilds on a street plan modeled after Washington, D.C.
1813	Portsmouth, New Hampshire, loses 244 buildings to fire. The city requires new buildings to be built of brick with slate roofs.
1820	The Great Fire of Savannah, Georgia, reduces half of the city's structures to ashes.
1821	The Great Fire of Fayetteville, North Carolina, burns 500 structures, including the State House.
1829	Augusta, Georgia, loses hundreds of buildings to fire.
1835	The Second Great Fire of New York City spreads to 17 city blocks. The city implements fire codes and orders a new municipal water supply, the Old Croton Aqueduct.
1838	Charleston, South Carolina, suffers fire damage to more than 1,000 buildings.
1845	The Third Great Fire of New York City destroys 345 buildings. The fire is able to be confined because of fire codes implemented after the fire in 1835.
1845	The Great Fire of Pittsburgh, Pennsylvania, destroys more than 1,000 buildings, one-third of all city structures.
1849	St. Louis, Missouri, loses 430 buildings, 23 steamboats, and a dozen other boats to fire. The city creates new building codes and installs an extensive water and sewage system.
1851	San Francisco, California, loses approximately 2,000 buildings to fire.
1862	Troy, New York, loses 671 buildings to fire.
1866	Portland, Maine, loses its commercial district and hundreds of homes to fire, leaving 10,000 homeless.
1871	The Great Chicago Fire destroys 3.3 square miles of the city, kills 300 people, and leaves 100,000 homeless.
1872	The Great Fire of Boston, Massachusetts, destroys 776 buildings, rendering thousands homeless.
1901	The Great Fire of Jacksonville, Florida, destroys 2,368 buildings in 146 city blocks. The fire leaves seven persons dead and 10,000 homeless.
1902	The Great Conflagration of Paterson, New Jersey, burns 459 buildings, City Hall, and the Free Public Library and leaves more than 500 families homeless.
1904	The Great Baltimore [Maryland] Fire burns 1,545 buildings over 70 city blocks.
1906	San Francisco suffers an earthquake, but 90 percent of the damage occurs from fires from ruptured gas lines over the next several days. Damage includes the loss of 25,000 buildings in 490 city blocks. The city responds with new building codes.

after the fire, the *Boston Morning Journal* reported that 17 streets had been widened, the water mains increased in size, and 32 new hydrants were added.[14]

Water and Sewers

After the Civil War, the nation saw rapid immigration, westward expansion, and an increased demand for manufactured goods. Some industries required large volumes of water, such as canning, chemical production, iron and steel, meatpacking, and paper production. By the end of the century, industrial requirements exceeded 10 billion gallons of water per day.[7] Bringing sufficient amounts of water into urban areas for fire-fighting, street cleaning, and improving the quality of life was a challenge, particularly water safe for human consumption. Although the existence of pathogenic bacteria had yet to be proven, it was patently obvious that noxious and potentially infectious contaminants were undesirable in drinking water.

Before 1800, pit privies in urban areas emptied onto yards or open channels by the street. As populations grew, this system gave way to cesspools and dry privies with collection traps for human excreta. The traps needed to be emptied on a regular basis and the most logical place for disposal in urban areas without municipal removal services was the open space between buildings. Here, mounds of night soil would collect, removable only by shovel and bucket. In 1874, New York City contracted Francis Swift, a purveyor of night-soil removal services, to "secure, at a proper distance, a place where night-soil could be deposited."[15] City officials hoped the effort would reduce disease outbreaks, the odor problem could be controlled, and the quality of life for the city's residents would improve. Despite partially solving the problem, New York City continued to suffer from overflowing cesspools, the daily deposition of large quantities of animal manure, and waste from slaughterhouses and industries that contaminated city streets and cisterns.

Sewers developed in urban America in a helter-skelter fashion with early ones consisting of hollowed out logs, which were sometimes, but not always, installed on a grade so they would channel runoff downslope into a nearby body of water. When water closets became available and populations consumed more water, it became clear that municipalities would have to own and maintain their own sewer systems for stormwater and sanitary waste. Not everyone was enamored of the water closet, however. In 1869, chemist Edward C.C. Stamford noted:

> It merely removes the bulk of our excreta from our houses to choke our rivers with foul deposits and rot at our neighbors' door. It introduces into our houses a most deadly enemy.[15]

Sewer gas was the deadly enemy. Water closets usually had undersized vents that clogged up, particularly with ice during the winter. The solution came after World War I when the modern flush toilet with a built-in trap to prevent gases from re-entering the room became widely available and affordable.

The first comprehensive sewer systems in the United States combined stormwater with industrial and sanitary waste into a single large-diameter conduit that drained into a nearby waterway (Brooklyn, New York, in 1855; Chicago in 1856; and Jersey City, New Jersey, in 1859).[16] Sewer systems that would manage stormwater and wastewater separately did not develop until later in the 19th century, a shift that did not come without controversy. The controversy can be traced to physician John Snow's classic mortality study of the 1854 cholera outbreak in London. That study showed that future outbreaks could be prevented by drawing water from a point upstream of any sewage discharge, filtered or not.[17] Snow's findings were not lost on civil engineers, nor were they lost on public health and municipal officials in both Europe and the United States. Public health officials began advocating separate wastewater and stormwater collection systems almost immediately. Their demands were challenged by civil engineers who believed that dumping raw sewage into water bodies was acceptable because the running water diluted the effluent and significantly removed health threats. Otherwise put, "The solution to pollution is dilution." Boards of health, dominated by physicians, clashed with civil engineers over the dilution issue, particularly as it affected downstream users. In response, the engineers recommended the most cost-effective solution—that downstream communities become responsible for filtering their own potable water at the point of intake.

The first city in the United States to use a slow sand filter process to clean its potable water supply was Poughkeepsie, New York, in 1874. By 1890, the Massachusetts Board of Health reported that sand filtration was effective in reducing the number of typhoid and cholera outbreaks. It took only a few short decades for most U.S. cities to have separate systems for handling their sanitary and stormwater, but the policy of dumping raw sewage and making downstream communities responsible for filtering their own potable water persisted.

The first use of chlorine to continually disinfect a municipal water supply in the United States began in 1908, at the Boonton Reservoir serving Jersey City. The use of chlorination also generated controversy, yet the process was rapidly installed in drinking water systems in many major U.S. cities to protect the public's health.[18] The controversy over chlorinating potable water has not receded with time. As recently as 2016, *Scientific American* questioned whether chlorination's benefits are outweighed by the link between exposure to chlorine and select cancers.[19]

The provision of clean water and efficient sewers to remove runoff (along with street cleaning measures) and sanitary sewage made a significant impact on reducing mortality rates by half in U.S. cities between the late 19th and early 20th centuries. One estimate of the "social rate of return" for investing in water and sewage technologies was greater than 23 to 1.[20] As concern over outbreaks of typhoid and cholera disappeared, other problems related to urban life became of more concern.

Housing

The Industrial Revolution was a catalyst for urban growth as new businesses located in cities to access the labor force and transportation hubs they needed to prosper. With prosperity, the moneyed class in New York City moved uptown, away from their middle-class row homes located near warehouses and factories, particularly on the Lower East Side. The modest three- to four-story row homes that the well-to-do left behind, along with any other vacant buildings, were quickly repurposed into smaller units with windowless internal rooms with no ventilation.

The laboring workforce needed places to sleep between shifts, and they rented whatever space they could. Unscrupulous landlords constructed five- to seven-story rental structures, often by adding stories to the existing row homes. The result was poorly constructed tenements, typically 25-feet wide by 100-feet long, with little space between them. These structures were prone to collapse, and sanitation was limited to communal water taps and badly maintained privies.

In 1845, physician John H. Griscom, the City Inspector of New York, published *The Sanitary Condition of the Laboring Population of New York*.[21] Griscom argued for housing reform and sanitation (a clean water supply, a sewage system, and street cleaning) and was the first to use the phrase "how the other half lives." He wrote of the abominable conditions suffered by tenement residents, especially those living in basements, but it took two decades before the State of New York responded to pressures from the daily newspapers and finally passed the Tenement House Act of 1867. That act defined a tenement as any rented residence with more than three families living independently and doing their own cooking, or by more than two families on a floor with common halls, stairways, yards, water closets, or privies. It prohibited basement apartments unless the ceiling was one foot above street level and also required one water closet per 20 residents, fire escapes, and some space between buildings to provide ventilation. What the act did not do was provide for strong enforcement mechanisms.[22]

Enter Jacob Riis. Danish-born Riis experienced immigrant life in New York City first hand. Riis's job as a police reporter brought him into the filth and crime of the Lower East Side on a regular basis and he was particularly adept at capturing photographic images of the conditions of the tenements. In 1890 he published his remarkable photos in *How the Other Half Lives*,[23] along with hard facts to stun his readers. They learned, for example, that 12 adults slept in a room only 13 feet across and that the death rate in New York City was higher than that for London, England, as well as for other major American cities (see Table 1.3).

Table 1.3. Statistics Bearing on the Tenement Problem in Major Cities

City	Population		Persons per Dwelling	Deaths		Death Rate	
	1880	1889	1880	1880	1889	1880	1889
New York, New York	1,206,229	1,575,073	16.37	31,937	39,679	26.47	25.19
London, England	3,816,483	4,351,738	7.90	81,431	75,683	21.30	17.40
Philadelphia, Pennsylvania	846,980	1,040,245	5.79	17,711	20,536	20.91	19.70
Brooklyn, New York	566,689	814,505	9.11	13,222	18,288	23.33	22.50
Boston, Massachusetts	362,535	420,000	8.26	8,612	10,259	23.75	24.42

Source: Reprinted from Jacob Riis, 1890.[23]

Contemporaneously with Riis, housing reformers such as Lawrence Veiller agitated to prohibit the construction of "dumbbell" tenements (deep but narrow buildings pinched in the middle so that each unit would have a window). The dumbbell design was seriously flawed because the distance between buildings at the ends was too tight for ready access. The pinched-in areas filled with garbage that was impossible to clean out, leading to both stench and vermin problems. The design was also dangerous because the pinched-in areas served as flues. When fires broke out, these structures became firetraps. Veiller also advocated toilets in every tenement and cried out for systematic enforcement of housing regulations. His efforts culminated in success when New York passed the Tenement House Act of 1901. Veiller then created a model regulatory law based on that act and distributed it to other cities across the United States, encouraging that it be adopted.[24]

Despite housing reforms, urban populations remained woefully crowded, living in tenements interspersed with industrial facilities and overt signs of massive growth (Figure 1.2). Those wishing to experience an old-style tenement building can visit the Lower East Side Tenement Museum, located at 97 Orchard Street in Manhattan. The 1863 building originally contained 22 apartments and a basement-level saloon. The building opened as a museum in 1988 and has since been designated a National Historic Site.[26]

Separation of the Professions

The Industrial Revolution brought with it demands for water, energy, transportation, and labor. It gave back industrial pollution and poor sanitary conditions. In the early years, architects and city planners worked with physicians with the understanding that human health and urban quality of life were intertwined. In the days before the causes of infectious diseases were understood, there could be no other logical explanation. As knowledge in both science and engineering grew, and as cities exploded with unmanageable growth and political corruption, the professions began to drift apart.

The first profession to separate itself from others was architecture. A group of architects in New York City incorporated in 1857 to define themselves as distinct from members of the building trades. By 1887, the American Institute of Architects had chapters in Albany, New York; Baltimore, Maryland; Boston, Massachusetts; Chicago, Illinois; Cincinnati, Ohio; Indianapolis, Indiana; Philadelphia, Pennsylvania; Providence, Rhode Island; San Francisco, California; St. Louis, Missouri; and Washington, D.C.[27]

Around that same time, physicians were beginning to set their target on improving public health. Before the Civil War, four National Sanitary Conventions were held in Philadelphia, Baltimore, New York, and Boston, all focused on quarantine. Interested physicians met in Atlantic City, New Jersey, in 1872 and created the American Public Health Association (APHA). Dr. Henry Bowditch summed up their efforts and those of other physicians in the emerging specialty of preventive medicine in his 1876 address to

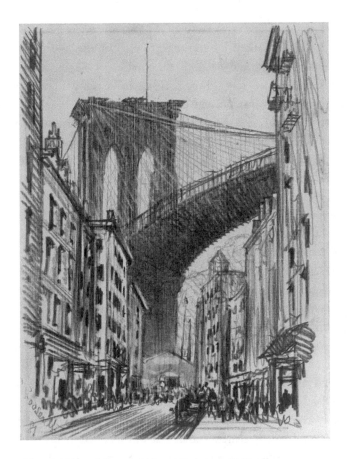

Source: Reprinted from the Library of Congress Prints and Photographs Division.[25]
Note: Originally published in Van Dyke JC. The New New York. New York, NY: The Macmillan Company, 1909.

Figure 1.2. Tenements Under the Brooklyn Bridge, Drawn by Joseph Pennell

the International Medical Congress in Philadelphia. Bowditch declared it time "to unravel the primal causes of all disease with the object of preventing it."[28] Today, APHA's Web site states that it "champions the health of all people in all communities" and lists its membership as more than 25,000 public health practitioners and academics worldwide.[29]

The APHA drew more than physician interest. Landscape architect Frederick Law Olmsted joined the organization in 1872, later chairing a committee on the relationship of shade trees, parks, and forests to public health.[30] Landscape architects believed that proximity to nature was necessary for human health and designed urban parks to provide places of escape from the filth and crowding of urban life. Central Park in New York City and Elm Park in Worchester, Massachusetts, are the gold standard for such efforts and remain a major source of recreation and civic pride for their urban populations today. The common interests of landscape architects crystalized in the founding of the

American Society of Landscape Architects in 1899. That association now represents more than 15,000 members nationwide according to the Web site.[31]

As the 19th century moved into the 20th, the professions became more even more specific in their respective practices. Civil engineers improved water treatment and sewage removal systems so that American cities with populations of more than 100,000 (Baltimore, Maryland; Cincinnati, Ohio; Cleveland, Ohio; Detroit, Michigan; Jersey City, New Jersey; Louisville, Kentucky; Milwaukee, Wisconsin; New Orleans, Louisiana; Philadelphia, Pennsylvania; Pittsburgh, Pennsylvania; St. Louis, Missouri.) instituted water filtration, chlorination, or both by 1916. The only exception was Memphis, Tennessee, which began both systems in 1936.[20] Unfortunately, clean, potable water was often transported by lead supply lines, with the major cities of New York, Chicago, Philadelphia, St. Louis, and Boston using them, at least in part, by 1900.[32] Lead in municipal water was not to be recognized as a public health hazard for decades, and in some instances the risk was denied well into the 21st century (e.g., Washington, D.C., in 2004; Flint, Michigan, in 2015).

The tools available for fighting infectious diseases in the early 1900s were limited. With cholera and typhoid controlled through sanitation, public health moved its focus to other causes of urban mortality, particularly tuberculosis and infant mortality. These were not diseases that could be controlled by either civil engineering or urban planning. The cure for tuberculosis before the advent of antibiotics was considered to be fresh air, good nutrition, and rest. Thus, scores of sanitariums (also known as sanatoriums or sanitaria) were established to provide places for recovery for sufferers of tuberculosis (known at the time as phthisis or consumption). Most sanitariums were small, often 20 beds in a large house away from the city center. The largest was founded in 1915—the Chicago Municipal Tuberculosis Sanitarium, with 950 beds.[33] Sanitariums served as a form of semi-quarantine, often for the select few who could pay for their services. As these facilities could not handle the large numbers of cases among the urban poor, the disease was not controlled in the United States until streptomycin, the first antibacterial agent effective against *Mycobacterium tuberculosis*, was developed in 1944.

Public health was better armed for attacking infant mortality than it was for tuberculosis. A leader in this regard was physician Sara Josephine Baker. Baker opened her medical practice in New York City in 1899, becoming a medical inspector for the city to augment her practice income. Shortly afterward she became the city's assistant commissioner of health and, in 1908, the first director of New York's Bureau of Child Hygiene. Baker's efforts focused on disease prevention and health education, particularly on basic hygiene for immigrants living in the poorest neighborhoods of New York City such as Hell's Kitchen and the Lower East Side. She created the Little Mothers League to train young girls to care for their infant siblings while their parents worked. She also championed clean milk stations to reduce infant diarrhea, as well as demanding the training and regulation of midwives. Baker's tireless efforts worked so that by 1923 New York City had the lowest infant mortality rate of any major city in America.[34] Today Baker is known as a public health reformer and child advocate. She earned a DrPH degree as well as an MD, and she published five books, 50 journal articles, and more than 200 popular pieces on preventive medicine.[35]

Urban planners had some internal struggles to overcome before they defined themselves through a separate professional organization. Most histories of urban planning begin with the Chicago World's Fair of 1893, with innovations that spawned the creation of the City Beautiful Movement. The fair made extensive use of streetlights and gleaming white building facades that stirred the imaginations of architects, landscape architects, and city planners alike. It encouraged architects to promote beauty and grand design for emerging cities, and landscape architects to promote harmony with nature along with monuments that would encourage civic pride. City planners (who were often also civil engineers) were encouraged to create comprehensive city designs that would improve both city beauty and functionality.

A widely cited text about the importance of the beautiful city appeared in 1901 by Charles M. Robinson. *The Improvement of Towns and Cities: Or, The Practical Basis of Civic Aesthetics*[36] encouraged private organizations to contract with planners to create beautiful city plans for rapidly growing urban America.[37] In 1902, the U.S. Senate approved the McMillan Plan, a beautiful city plan designed to update Pierre Charles L'Enfant's original plan for the nation's capital (see Chapter 2). The McMillan Plan is still in place, with the document available online for the public to peruse.[38] The plan called for much of what is experienced by visitors to Washington, D.C., today, including the site of a relocated rail terminal, the parks system, a redesigned mall, and many monuments to showcase national pride.

At the same time that the City Beautiful Movement was strengthening, the Progressive Movement was taking hold. Progressives, such as Riis and Baker, believed in social justice—that social problems (e.g., disease, poverty, class warfare, racism, and violence) could be addressed by education and by providing better living and working conditions, particularly for urban populations. A rising activist in the Progressive Movement was Benjamin Marsh, a social worker and secretary to the New York City Committee on Congestion of Population. In 1908, Marsh organized an exhibition on city planning at the American Museum of Natural History with an emphasis on overcrowding as the roots of poverty, poor health, and crime. The exhibition was popular, drawing about 50,000 visitors.[37] Determined to place social reforms at the root of city planning, Marsh proceeded to write book on the topic, *An Introduction to City Planning; Democracy's Challenge to the American City,* which he self-published in early 1909.[39]

With his newly claimed identity as a city planner, Marsh attended the First National Conference on City Planning in Washington, D.C., shortly after his book appeared. He pushed hard at that conference for attendees to focus on social reforms, perhaps too hard. His firebrand style led Frederick Law Olmsted, Jr., to take a more conservative position, asking for a resolution that would allow a second conference to be held the following year on "comprehensive" city planning. Olmsted's goal was to include practitioners from all of the professions that participate in the planning process rather than let it be hijacked by Marsh.

At the second conference, Olmsted gave the opening address, stating that city planning was an emerging discipline that should seek "the connections which link the planning of all the diverse elements of the physical city together." He argued that the new discipline should not be a tool for social engineering, thus drawing support from architects, civil engineers, landscape architects, and even housing reform activists.[37] As a result, the second conference may have been the true beginning of urban planning as a fledgling discipline.

The first incorporated urban planning organization was the American City Planning Institute in 1917, renamed the American Institute of Planners (AIP) in 1939. The 1917 organization focused on advancing the science of the urban planning, electing Frederick Law Olmsted, Jr., as its first president. Additional professional and academic organizations representing urban planning are listed in Table 1.4. The largest of the professional planning organizations today is the American Planning Association, the result of a merger between the AIP and the American Society of Planning Officials in 1979.

Differences in Training

In the nation's early years, boards of health focused on controlling epidemics by quarantine, and both physicians and city planners tried to address the health of urban populations by improving the quality of water, sewage, and housing. Later,

Table 1.4. Professional Organizations and Select Events Related to the Development of Urban Planning: United States

Year	Organization
1852	The American Society of Civil Engineers is founded.
1857	The American Institute of Architects is founded.
1898	The First International Urban Planning Conference is held in New York City.
1899	The American Society of Landscape Architects is founded.
1906	The American Society of Sanitary Engineers is founded.
1909	The First National Conference on City Planning takes place in Washington, D.C.
1910	The Second National Conference on City Planning takes place in Rochester, New York.
1917	The American City Planning Institute is founded, becoming the American Institute of Planners (AIP) in 1939.
1934	The American Society of Planning Officials (ASPO) is founded.
1959	The Association of Collegiate Schools of Planning is founded (http://www.acsp.org).
1960	The National Education Development Committee of the AIP is created to credential planning program graduates (1977 first AIP exam).
1978	American Planning Association is founded from a merger of the AIP and the ASPO (https://www.planning.org).
1978	American Institute of Certified Planners (AICP) is founded. AICP Certification is introduced (https://www.planning.org/aicp).

architects and landscape and city planners encouraged new urban designs that would provide contact with nature, engender civic pride, and improve the function of the city. Public health practitioners encouraged the practice of preventive medicine, with a focus on immunization, health education, and screening programs. With differences in the professions becoming more apparent each year, it was only natural that they found separate homes for the academic training of future practitioners, a move that would solidify their differences. Specifically, Harvard claims to have started the first urban planning program (1900) and Johns Hopkins founded the first School of Hygiene and Public Health with funding from the Rockefeller Foundation (1916).

As the professions continued to drift apart, their respective graduate programs expanded to fill what were perceived to be specialized needs. Public health created training divisions in behavioral science and health education, biostatistics, environmental health, epidemiology, and health services management and policy. Urban planning offered training in housing and community development, environmental and land use planning, economic and regional development, historic preservation, transportation planning, urban design, and geographic information systems. The development of public health as a separate field is demonstrated by the events in Table 1.5.

The professional organizations representing their respective fields helped create accreditation criteria for the academic programs, as well as developing certification examinations for practitioners in some of the subfields. Today, the Planning Accreditation Board (PAB) accredits North American schools and programs in urban planning, and the Council for Education in Public Health (CEPH) accredits those for public health. A review of the standards and criteria for accrediting these training programs shows that the word "health" does not appear anywhere in PAB documentation[40] and "urban planning" does not appear in the standards and criteria for CEPH.[41] Perhaps the closest acknowledgment that urban planners share any overlap in mission with public health appears in the "Values and Ethics" section of the PAB standards and criteria document, which lists "an appreciation of natural resource and pollution control factors in planning, and understanding of how to create sustainable futures."[40]

Paradigm Shifts

For at least the first two-thirds of the 20th century, most American urban planners were champions of low-density suburban development with tree-lined cul-de-sacs and shiny new shopping malls. Cities and towns were in decline, with their main streets pockmarked with boarded-up storefronts while the suburbs expanded at breakneck speed. These changes were decried by Jane Jacobs, a journalist and activist who espoused the virtues of living in the chaos of a vibrant urban neighborhood.

Table 1.5. Professional Organizations and Select Events Related to the Development of Public Health: United States

Year	Organization
1798	Congress passes the Marine Hospital Service (MHS) Act, the first federally funded disease prevention agency. The MHS was the genesis for the eventual development of the U.S. Public Health Service.
1872	The American Public Health Association was founded to "advocate for adoption of scientific advances relevant to public health and to support public education to improve community health" (https://www.apha.org).
1884	The National Conference of State Boards of Health begins meeting annually, later to incorporate as the Association of State and Territorial Health Officials in 1942 (http://www.astho.org).
1937	The National Environmental Health Association was founded to "establish a standard of excellence for the developing environmental health profession" (http://www.neha.org). Credentials offered: • Certified in Comprehensive Food Safety • Certified Environmental Health Technician • Certified Installers of On-site Wastewater Treatment Systems • Certified Professional—Food Safety • Healthy Homes Specialist • Registered Environmental Health Specialist/Registered Sanitarian • Additional programs in hazardous substances training
1938	The National Conference of Governmental Industrial Hygienists holds its first meeting, becoming the American Conference of Governmental Industrial Hygienists in 1946. The goal was for hygienists in the public sector to "define the science of occupational and environmental health" (http://www.acgih.org).
1939	The American Industrial Hygiene Association is founded for "non-physicians dedicated to improving worker health" (https://www.aiha.org).
1941	The Association of Schools of Public Health is founded becoming the Association of Schools and Programs of Public Health in 2013 (http://www.aspph.org).
1950	The Society for Public Health Education is founded to "promote healthy behaviors, healthy communities, and healthy environments" (http://www.sophe.org).
1960	The American Board of Industrial Hygiene is founded for credentialing industrial hygienists (http://www.abih.org). Credential offered: • Certified Industrial Hygienist
1974	Council on Education for Public Health is established to accredit schools and programs in public health (http://ceph.org).
1978	A National Task Force on the Preparation and Practice of Health Educators is established, incorporating as the National Commission for Health Education Credentialing in 1988 (http://www.nchec.org). Credentials offered: • Certified Health Education Specialist • Master Certified Health Education Specialist
1992	The National Association of Local Boards of Health is established to give a national voice to local boards of health (http://www.nalboh.org).
2005	The National Board of Public Health Examiners is established to certify the skills and knowledge base of public health professionals (http://www.nbphe.org/aboutthecph.cfm). Credential offered: • Certified in Public Health
2007	The Public Health Accreditation Board is established to accredit tribal, state, local, and territorial public health departments (http://www.phaboard.org).

Jacobs published *The Death and Life of Great American Cities* in 1961, presenting a damning view of urban planning practices that pushed both suburbanization and slum clearance (urban renewal). Instead, she espoused city planning that focused on

- "Mixed primary uses" that would bring people into the streets at different times of the day.
- Short blocks to encourage pedestrian use.
- Buildings of varying ages and states of repair to generate interest.
- Density.[42]

Both academic and practicing planners alike scorned Jacobs's ideas. She was dismissed as too much of a firebrand without training in the planning profession, much as Marsh had been half a century before. Her ideas, however, left an indelible mark on the planning profession as over the next few decades suburban life degenerated into urban sprawl with ugly strip malls and traffic woes for commuters. The realities of auto-dependent living meant that access to civil, health, and recreational services were restricted for children, the disabled, the elderly, and the poor who did not have ready access to transportation. Restrictive zoning practices also concentrated undesirable land uses in select neighborhoods where air and water pollution were increased, raising issues of environmental equity and justice.

By the 1980s it became obvious that urban planning needed a new plan. That new plan was the New Urbanism movement, encouraging urban designs that would result in walkable, mixed-use neighborhoods with accessible public institutions and local shopping. Anyone wishing to experience one or more of the early New Urbanist designs might consider visiting the communities of Baldwin Park (outside Orlando, Florida) or Seaside (west of Panama City, Florida).

The New Urbanism movement was solidified in 1993 with the founding of the Congress for the New Urbanism (CNU).[43] That organization continues to host an annual national meeting, as well as an online journal to share its ideas and mission. What is different about CNU membership is that it is not restricted to members of the planning profession. Membership is open to anyone who designs, builds, or advocates for better urban living, regardless of his or her training or affiliation. The New Urbanism movement also succeeded in broadening academic urban planning, with new topics such as "brownfields redevelopment," "green building," "sustainability," "traditional neighborhood development," and "transit-oriented development" becoming incorporated into traditional urban planning curricula.

Public health concerns also shifted after mid-century. They now focused on access to medical care and the skyrocketing costs of treating chronic diseases. The public was concerned about AIDS, cancer, diabetes, heart disease, and stroke, and a baby boom generation that was likely to drive health care costs even higher as they aged. In 1979, Surgeon General Julius Richmond issued a landmark report entitled *Healthy People: The Surgeon General's Report on Health Promotion and Disease Prevention.*[44] The report made a strong statement about individuals taking personal responsibility for their own health by practicing responsible behaviors, ensuring proper nutrition, and getting regular physical exercise. The Healthy People initiative continues in the United States today, essentially rewritten with new goals and objectives for the nation's health each decade. *Healthy People 2020* sets out three goals: (1) attain high-quality, longer lives free of preventable disease, disability, injury, and premature death; (2) achieve health equity, eliminate disparities, and improve the health of all groups; and (3) create social and physical environments that promote good health for all.

The World Health Organization (WHO) began stressing an ecological view of health during the 1980s, recognizing that "Health is created and lived by people within the settings of their everyday life."[45] In 1992, the WHO Centre for Health Development was created in Kobe, Japan (WHO-Kobe Centre or WKC), with a vision statement: "Health for all in urban environments."[46] This vision is apt as the WKC estimates that 70 percent of the world's population will be living in cities by 2050 and the speed of urbanization is rapidly outpacing the development of infrastructure, services, and other resources. As urban planning plays a distinct role in creating healthy, equitable, and sustainable cities, the WKC has a Web page on healthy urban planning, noting that WKC works to

- Build evidence of the impact of urban planning on health equity.
- Adapt urban planning tools to promote health equity.
- Document specific experiences of urban planning interventions aimed on health equity, and derive lessons for policymakers.[46]

Despite what seems to have been obvious to those creating the WKC in the early 1990s, the links between urban planning and public health in the United States were broken. In fact, Greenberg and colleagues[47] investigated the links between city planning and public health in the United States by reviewing both the primary literature and graduate programs in the respective fields from 1978 through 1990. Their results found little overlap and called for the fields to re-establish their common cause.

Bringing the fields back together has not been an easy task, nor is it complete. Northridge and colleagues[48] reported that the New Urbanism devoted more time to creating linkages to public health than vice versa. Part of this may be because planners in general and New Urbanists in particular are visionaries by nature. They understand the importance of the social context of community and can readily categorize neighborhoods and the built environment. New Urbanists tend to easily equate a healthy city as synonymous with healthy people and a good quality of life.

In contrast, public health and preventive medicine professionals focus on identifying diseases and instituting preventive measures and treatments that have been demonstrated to be efficacious. These dedicated practitioners are very much concerned with protecting the public from misguided practices that might do more harm than good, both immediately and in the long term. In line with the practice of demanding scientific proof (evidence-based outcomes), the Healthy People initiative requires that each health objective be benchmarked with data and monitored for progress toward a preset goal, often a decade away.

Some of the social determinants of disease, such as economic stability, education status, and the impacts of racism are difficult to measure. It took time for public health researchers, particularly social epidemiologists, to build new databases and analyze the relationships between the social determinants of health and particular health outcomes. When the *Healthy People 2020* initiative was launched in 2010, it included, for the first time, linking the social determinants of disease to the overarching goal of achieving social and physical environments that "promote good health for all."[49] Other signs that the professions are reconnecting, finding common ground if not their original roots, are found in Table 1.6.

Table 1.6. Signs of Urban Planning and Public Health Reconnecting

Year	Signs of Relinking the Professions
1999	The World Health Organization releases *Healthy Cities and the City Planning Process*, encouraging planners to develop health as a key principle in urban planning.[50]
2003	The Institute of Medicine publishes *The Future of the Public's Health in the 21st Century*, with a separate section on the social determinants of health.[51]
2003	The *American Journal of Public Health* publishes a special issue linking public health and planning (September).
2003	The *American Journal of Health Promotion* publishes a special issue linking public health and planning (September).
2003	The *Journal of Urban Health* publishes a special issue linking public health and planning (December).
2005	The *Journal of Urban Health* publishes a special issue linking public health and planning (February).
2006	The *Journal of the American Planning Association* publishes a special issue linking public health and planning (Winter).
2009	The Pew Charitable Trust and the Robert Wood Johnson Foundation launch their joint Health Impact Project that promotes "the use of health impact assessments to incorporate health into decisions made by sectors—such as transportation, planning, education or housing—that do not traditionally focus on health outcomes."[52]
2010	The *Healthy People 2020* initiative is launched, including the social determinants of disease for the first time.[49]
2010	The Robert Wood Johnson Foundation issues a landmark document addressing vulnerable populations. That report concluded, "Health starts where we live, learn, work and play."[52]
2011	The National Research Council releases *Improving Health in the United States: The Role of Health Impact Assessment* indicating: "An infield—health impact assessment (HIA)—can assist decision-makers in examining the potential health effects of proposed projects, programs, plans, policies."[53]
2000-Present	Hundreds of articles that link public health and urban planning are published sporadically by various peer-reviewed journals. Common topics include active living, aging, air and water quality, climate change, crime and violence, food security, housing, noise, obesity, social environments, sprawl, traffic congestion, transportation access, walking and cycling, and more.

Sharing Tools and Skill Sets—Summary of the Chapters

It is vitally important for planning and public health practitioners who are trained in very different ways to learn to understand what each profession brings to the table so they can work together to improve the health of their communities. To this end, Chapters 2 and 3 define and describe the building blocks of each of the professions, their major areas of expertise, and their professional ethics and advocacy roles.

Specifically, Chapter 2 begins with the planning profession, noting that planners gather information from stakeholders in both the public and private sectors, and generate projects that address local and regional needs. Planning training covers land use, economic development, housing and community development, and other fields such as design and transportation—elements that are all important for creating healthy and vibrant communities.

Chapter 3 continues with the development of the public health profession. Public health practitioners envision communities where everyone lives a life free of preventable disease, disability, injury, and premature death. The profession uses the tools of surveillance and epidemiology to identify and intercede in health problems; the tools of environmental health to help create healthy national, regional, and local environments; and advocacy to make changes that benefit the health and well-being of us all.

Chapter 4 provides the context for the remaining chapters in the book. It identifies the tools that members of both professions can use either separately or, preferably, jointly, to help solve problems in their communities. Some of the tools might be familiar, but it is likely that many others are not—perhaps considered beyond the realm of expertise for some. In either case, we suggest that by becoming familiar with the terminology surrounding the tools, if not the nuts and bolts of their use, professionals in both professions can work together more effectively. The knowledge should bring respect to the outcomes-driven community processes that these tools encourage.

Chapters 5 through 10 contain explanations about the tools, along with case studies that illustrate the use of each one. To make the chapters easy to follow, we organized them first to address basic local challenges (Chapter 5) and progressed to complex regional ones (Chapter 9), ending in the indoor environment in Chapter 10. Presentations of the case studies benefit from our having been involved in following them, sometimes intimately and sometimes only tangentially. Regardless of our level of personal involvement, we feel they are worthy of your perusal as they might spark comparisons to problems in your own locale.

Chapter 5 covers three tools that should interest professionals in both planning and public health: checklists, information gathering/public outreach, and health impact assessments. These are relatively simple tools likely to be useful in all communities, large and small. Two local health impact assessments are presented as case studies. The first describes a county-scale effort to repurpose an abandoned rail line. The goals for the project included providing opportunities for increased physical activity that were both accessible and safe in a moderately urbanized area, and improving both social cohesion and the local economy. The second case study considers options for traffic calming along an artery traversing several urban communities. Here the goal was to reduce collisions with pedestrians, bicyclists, and drivers, as well as noise and pollution. Economic impacts and access to transit, healthy food, and other services were also taken into consideration.

The tools presented in Chapter 6 include accessing and interpreting population data, mapping as communication about the population at risk, and hazard mitigation analysis. We recognize that both professions can claim expertise in the use of the first two of the tools; however, we point out nuances that may escape some recent advocates of their use. By contrast, the third tool, hazard mitigation analysis, is likely to be new to many planning and public health professionals. The case study in this chapter explains the use of the tools at three geographic scales: the State of Texas, the Houston–Galveston region, and Galveston City.

Chapter 7 covers social network analysis, environmental justice assessment, and political process assessment. Two California cases demonstrate the use of these tools relative to legal and moral obligations of both government and the private sector. The first case study tackles the problems faced by homeless veterans, including their mental and physical health, as well as employment challenges. The second case study takes on the thorny issue of food security in the greater Los Angeles area. Food security is complex. It is not only about educating the public about nutrition, nor is it only about providing sufficient amount of food for families. It also includes making nutritious options available to the population through tools that planners primarily use, such as zoning and various types of economic incentives for attracting quality farm, retail, and restaurant food options.

Deciding to redevelop a seriously contaminated site requires collaborative problem solving, planning and design charrettes, and risk analysis. Chapter 8 describes these tools and how they were applied in a case study the Fernald Nuclear Weapon Site outside Cincinnati. It was clear that the site would never be remediated to its background levels before being used for nuclear weapons production for three decades. The case study addresses the question: how safe is safe enough?

One of the largest issues we have encountered is presented in Chapter 9—the situation in which proponents of a major regional asset may face stakeholders who oppose the project. The chapter addresses how to bring project boosters and those holding a "not-in-my-backyard" (NIMBY) stance into collaborations that inform the decision-making process. The tools covered in this, our most complex chapter, include environmental impact statements, regional economic impact analysis, and cost and benefit analysis. Two case studies using these tools come to very different decisions—that of the Denver International Airport and the construction of a liquefied natural gas plant at Sparrows Point, Maryland.

Chapter 10 covers the indoor environment where the overwhelming majority of us spend more than 90 percent of our time. We review the historic and current rules under which we select locations for land uses and how these codes require that built structures are at least minimally protective of human health and safety. Focusing on the challenging issue of indoor air quality, the chapter concludes with two case studies in New Orleans. There, green building practitioners are working to improve the health of indoor environments while reducing demands on resources.

Finally, Chapter 11 summarizes how we keep abreast of changes and opportunities in our professional fields. As academics in a professional school that cross-pollinates the fields of planning and public health, it is only natural for us to assume that the two professions should work closely together. We recognize, however, that planning and public health departments in the real (nonacademic) world rarely share the same benefits of cross-pollination. Thus, we hope that the tools provided in the case study chapters will help both health officials and planners to assess and manage 21st-century challenges in new ways that stretch their traditional limits. We also hope our efforts provide a refreshed vocabulary that helps the professions better communicate and respect each other's strengths.

References

1. Preston SH. Human mortality throughout history and prehistory. In: Simon JL, ed. *The State of Humanity*. London, England: Blackwell Publishing Professional; 1994.

2. Bumgarner JR. *The Health of the Presidents: The 41 United States Presidents Through 1993 From a Physician's Point of View*. Jefferson, NC: McFarland; 1994.

3. Pyle GF. The diffusion of cholera in the United States in the nineteenth century. *Geogr Anal*. 2010;1(1):59–75.

4. Library of Congress Prints and Photographs Division. Drawing by Frank H. Taylor, 1895. The Lazaretto, Delaware River vicinity, Essington, Delaware County, PA. Available at: http://www.loc.gov/pictures/item/pa0415.photos.133644p/resource. Accessed March 22, 2017.

5. Lazaretto Quarantine Station. 2010. Available at: http://www.ushistory.org/laz/history/index.htm. Accessed January 3, 2016.

6. Shattuck L. *Report of the Sanitary Commission of Massachusetts 1850*. Boston, MA: Dutton & Wentworth, State Printers; 1850.

7. Dworsky L. *The Nation and Its Water Resources*. US Public Health Service; 1962.

8. *Historical Statistics of the United States: 1789–1945*. Washington, DC: US Census Bureau; 1949.

9. Tarr JA, McCurley III J, McMichael FC, Yosie T. Water and wastes: a retrospective assessment of wastewater technology in the United States, 1800–1932. *Technol Cult*. 1984;25(2):226–263.

10. Shelhamer C. How fire disaster shaped the evolution of the New York City Building Code. *ICC Build Saf J [Online]*. December 14, 2010. Available at: http://bsj.iccsafe.org/2010Dec/features/nyc_code_history.html. Accessed March 14, 2017.

11. Miller D. *City of the Century; The Epic of Chicago and the Making of America*. New York, NY: Simon and Schuster; 1996.

12. Olmsted FL. Chicago in distress. *The Nation*. November 9, 1871. Available at: http://www.greatchicagofire.org/media-event-library/chicago-distress. Accessed December 30, 2015.

13. Schons M. The Chicago Fire of 1871 and the "Great Rebuilding." National Geographic Education. 2011. Available at: http://education.nationalgeographic.org/news/chicago-fire-1871-and-great-rebuilding. Accessed December 29, 2015.

14. One year after Boston's Great Fire of 1872. *Bost Morning J*. November 13, 1873;40.

15. Stamford E. The sewage question. In: Trowbridge J, ed. *Annual of Scientific Discovery*. Boston, MA: Gould and Lincoln; 1870:72–73.

16. Metcalf L, Eddy HP. *Design of Sewers*. 2nd ed. New York, NY: McGraw-Hill Company; 1928.

17. Snow J. *On the Mode of Communication of Cholera*. London, England: John Churchill; 1855.

18. Hazen A. *Clean Water and How to Get It*. 2nd ed. New York, NY: John Wiley & Sons; 1914.

19. Tapped out?: Are chlorine's beneficial effects in drinking water offset by its links to cancer? *Scientific American*. 2016. Available at: http://www.scientificamerican.com/article/earth-talks-tapped-out. Accessed September 18, 2016.

20. Cutler D, Miller G. The role of public health improvements in health advances: the twentieth-century United States. *Demography*. 2005;42(1):1–22.

21. Griscom J. *The Sanitary Condition of the Laboring Population of New York*. New York, NY: Harper; 1845.

22. Plunz R. *History of Housing in New York City: Dwelling Type and Social Change in the American Metropolis*. New York, NY: Columbia University Press; 1990.

23. Riis JA. *How the Other Half Lives*. 1st ed. New York, NY: C. Scribner's Sons; 1890.

24. Lubove R. Lawrence Veiller and the New York State Tenement House Commission of 1900. *Mississippi Val Hist Rev*. 1961;47(4):659–677.

25. Library of Congress Prints and Photographs Division. Tenements under Brooklyn Bridge (Brooklyn Bridge tenements). Available at: http://www.loc.gov/pictures/item/2007665887. Accessed March 22, 2017.

26. Tenement Museum New York City. Available at: https://tenement.org. Accessed January 5, 2016.

27. The American Institute of Architects. History of the American Institute of Architects. Available at: http://www.aia.org/about/history/AIAB028819. Accessed January 6, 2016.

28. Bowditch H. Address on hygiene and preventive medicine. In: Ashhurst JJ, ed. *Transactions of the International Medical Congress of Philadelphia, 1876*. Philadelphia, PA: Collins, Printer for the Congress; 1877:21–48.

29. American Public Health Association. APHA Web site. Available at: https://www.apha.org. Accessed July 20, 2017.

30. Peterson JA. The impact of sanitary reform upon American urban planning, 1840–1890. *J Soc Hist*. 1979;13(1):83–103.

31. American Society of Landscape Architects. About us. Available at: https://advertise.asla.org/about-us. Accessed July 20, 2017.

32. Baker MN. *The Quest for Pure Water: The History of Water Purification From the Earliest Records to the Twentieth Century*. New York, NY: American Waterworks Association; 1949.

33. Sachs TB. Provision for infants in Chicago Municipal Tuberculosis Sanitarium. *JAMA*. 1915;64(1):72.

34. Morantz-Sanchez R. Sara Josephine Baker. In: Garraty JA, Carnes MC, eds. *American National Biography*. New York, NY: Oxford University Press; 1999:32–34.

35. Parry MS. Sara Josephine Baker (1873–1945). *Am J Public Health*. 2006;96(4):620–621.

36. Robinson CM. *The Improvement of Towns and Cities: Or, The Practical Basis of Civic Aesthetics*. New York, NY: G.P. Putnam's Sons; 1901.

37. Peterson JA. The birth of organized city planning in the United States, 1909–1910. *J Am Plan Assoc*. 2009;75(2):123–133.

38. The 1902 Report of the Senate Park Commission, Also Known as the McMillan Commission. Available at: http://www.nationalmall.net/resource/mcmillan.html. Accessed January 10, 2016.

39. Marsh BC, Ford GB. *An Introduction to City Planning: Democracy's Challenge to the American City*. New York, NY: Privately Printed; 1909.

40. *Planning Accreditation Board Accreditation Standards and Criteria*. Chicago, IL: Planning Accreditation Board; 2012.

41. *Council on Education in Public Health Accreditation Criteria and Procedures*. Washington, DC: Council on Education in Public Health; 2011.

42. Jacobs J. *The Death and Life of Great American Cities*. New York, NY: Random House; 1961.

43. Congress for the New Urbanism. 2015. Available at: https://www.cnu.org. Accessed January 15, 2016.

44. Healthy People 2020. About Healthy People. Available at: http://www.healthypeople.gov/2020/About-Healthy-People. Accessed January 18, 2016.

45. Ashton J, Grey P, Barnard K. Healthy cities—WHO's new public health initiative. *Health Promot Int*. 1986;1(3):319–324.

46. World Health Organization. Healthy urban planning. Available at: http://www.who.int/kobe_centre/interventions/urban_planning/en. Accessed January 12, 2016.

47. Greenberg MR, Popper FJ, West BM. The TOADS: a new American urban epidemic. *Urban Aff Rev.* 1990;25(3):435–454.

48. Northridge ME, Sclar ED, Biswas P. Sorting out the connections between the built environment and health: a conceptual framework for navigating pathways and planning healthy cities. *J Urban Health.* 2003;80(4):556–568.

49. Secretary's Advisory Committee on Health Promotion and Disease Prevention Objectives for 2020. Healthy People 2020: an opportunity to address societal determinants of health in the United States. 2010. Available at: http://www.healthypeople.gov/2010/hp2020/advisory/SocietalDeterminantsHealth.htm. Accessed January 16, 2016.

50. Duhl L, Kristin-Sanchez A. *Healthy Cities and the City Planning Process.* Copenhagen, Denmark: World Health Organization Regional Office for Europe; 1999.

51. Committee for the Study of the Future of Public Health. *The Future of Public Health.* Washington, DC: National Academies Press; 1988.

52. Health Impact Project. Pew Trusts and Robert Wood Johnson Foundation. 2009. Available at: http://www.pewtrusts.org/en/projects/health-impact-project. Accessed January 18, 2016.

53. National Research Council. *Improving Health in the United States.* Washington, DC: National Academies Press; 2011.

2

BUILDING BLOCKS OF URBAN PLANNING

Defining the Profession

The American Planning Association (APA) defines planning (urban planning, city planning, regional planning) as "a dynamic profession that works to improve the welfare of people and their communities by creating more convenient, equitable, healthful, efficient, and attractive places for present and future generations."[1] Planners gather information from stakeholders in both the public and private sectors and generate projects that address local and regional needs.

From the earliest beginnings of the profession, planners were concerned with the economic and physical growth of cities. Some were also concerned with promoting public health, social equity, and both aesthetics and a sense of place. Today's planners still hold these objectives, but they are also concerned about shrinking and dying cities (from lack of jobs, water shortages, flight to the suburbs), urban sprawl, traffic congestion, the regulatory environment, and what global warming will mean to us all. Their tools have advanced beyond the drafting tables and municipal meetings of the 19th century to include geographic information systems, complex modeling, physical and graphics design software packages, and the financial tools that allow creative public–private partnerships. Planners often create and host charrettes (facilitated planning workshops) to involve a diverse set of stakeholders in visioning the future for a particular locality or region. Charrettes also provide planners with stakeholder feedback to help ensure that any plan they put forward appropriately addresses the challenge at hand.

Planners in colonial America were commonly surveyors who were charged with laying out the plan for a new town, often with a commons, square, or marketplace at the center. The towns were usually situated where they would connect to the outside world for trade via a river, canal, or port. The British system of metes (a straight run distance along a compass bearing) and bounds (a boundary delineated by a natural or man-made marker) was generally used to describe the locations of parcels of land. This system, still used in England, allowed surveyors to take into account local topography and the physical boundaries described in original land grants, as well as in subsequent land transfers. The metes and bounds system had some limitations, however, as some of the physical markers described in land-related documents were not always permanent (watercourses moved, trees and coastal landmarks disappeared after storms, structures burned down). Thus, boundary disputes were fairly common.

After independence, surveyors were charged with using the Public Land Survey System (PLSS, the Rectangular Survey System, or the Township and Range System) to explore and map the nation's expanding western territories. The PLSS required surveyors to begin with a designated baseline (parallel of latitude) and a principle meridian. They then laid out six-by-six–mile townships (36 square miles) relative to those points. The one-square-mile sections within each township were subdivided into aliquot parts, ideally by quartering each section to yield four 160-acre divisions and then subdividing each of those to yield parcels of 40 acres. Roads were laid out one mile apart along section boundaries, with commercial uses often developing at arterial intersections. Travel would be a bit easier in major cities where the distance between intersecting roads could be reduced to one-half mile apart, but forward progress was still limited by only being able to go straight or at right angles. The effect of the PLSS can be readily seen by anyone peering out the window of an airplane flying over the United States at almost any point west of the Appalachian Mountains.

Engineers and architects planned not only for the physical growth of cities, but also for housing, parks, public buildings, and services such as sanitation and transportation. In 1791, President Washington appointed Pierre Charles L'Enfant to plan the nation's new capital city. Thomas Jefferson sent L'Enfant a letter outlining his limited task—to provide a drawing of suitable sites for the federal city and its public buildings. L'Enfant had a grand vision not only of a street grid and the locations of a few federal buildings but also of diagonally intersecting avenues that created circles and rectangular plazas where notable Americans could be honored with impressive monuments. The diagonal avenues would radiate from the highest point of land—Capitol Hill. Canals, parks, many stately buildings, and broad avenues would abound throughout the district. The president's house would be a monumental structure five times the size of the White House that was eventually constructed.

The commissioners charged with overseeing the planning effort considered the L'Enfant plan too grandiose and costly. When L'Enfant protested, insisting that the commissioners implement his entire design, they simply replaced him with surveyor Andrew Ellicott. Enlisting the aid of his brother Benjamin, Ellicott simplified the plan and sent it to printers in Philadelphia, Pennsylvania, so it could be published for wide circulation (Figure 2.1).

Other early planning efforts to improve the lives of city residents in the United States, as well as the controversies about how the profession should develop at the end of the 19th century, are described in Chapter 1. It took multiple national conferences on planning before the profession was able to launch its own organization, the American City Planning Institute, in 1917. By that time, the Model-T had already created the American love affair

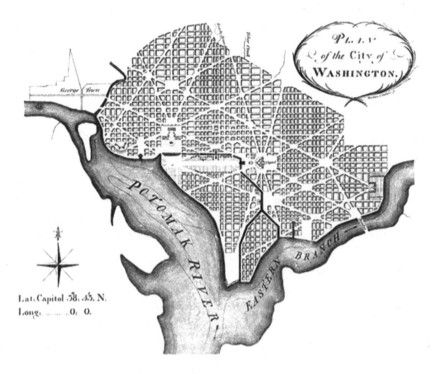

Source: Reprinted from the Library of Congress via Wikimedia Commons.[2]

Figure 2.1. Plan of the City of Washington, D.C., March 1792, by Andrew Ellicott, Revised From Pierre Charles L'Enfant

with the automobile; an individual in New York City could place a telephone call to someone in San Francisco, California; and new labor laws provided Americans with leisure time that allowed them to go to movie theaters and baseball games. The rapid growth of urban America led planners to the realization that states and municipalities not only needed to plan for urban growth but also needed a means to implement those plans.

Land Use

Land-use planning, regional planning, and urban planning are terms used to describe strategies used by governing authorities to define areas where specific types of land use may occur. The goal of land-use planning is to manage both the economic and physical growth of a region in an organized fashion, one that allows for both natural and man-made resources to be protected and, at least in theory, to minimize conflicts over competing land uses. One tool for obtaining the space to create the infrastructure needed to support controlled growth (for a regional airport, for instance) is the power of eminent domain. Other tools that planners use to restrict growth to select sectors or to transform the physical form of their communities are zoning practices, planned unit developments, and form-based codes.

Eminent Domain

The federal and state governments have the power of eminent domain, or the authority to take private property for the public good as long as just compensation is provided (codified as "The Takings Clause" of the Fifth Amendment to the U.S. Constitution). Federal use of eminent domain has often been used for siting public buildings (customs houses, postal facilities) and securing land or rights of way for large-scale infrastructure development (aqueducts and dams, highways, public utilities, and our national forest and park systems).[3]

States often exercise eminent domain for public works projects (reservoirs, bridges, and tunnels) or to protect natural resources (wetlands or fragile environments). They may also, by statutory authority, extend the power of eminent domain to the municipalities in their state. When localities use eminent domain for siting schools, libraries, or other municipal facilities, it is usually clear to everyone that the purpose of taking private property is for the public good. When municipalities exercise the power for the purposes of local economic development, however, questions may arise as to whether the taking truly serves the public good or whether it simply supports private interests.

For example, a 2005 U.S. Supreme Court decision recognized the authority of New London, Connecticut, to take non-blighted private property by eminent domain and to transfer that property for a dollar a year to a private developer to increase municipal revenues.[4] The public outcry from the court's decision was profound, leading President George W. Bush to issue Executive Order 13406 in 2006.[5] That order prevents the federal government from using the power of eminent domain for the "purpose of advancing the economic interest of private parties to be given ownership or use of the property taken." Although the executive order restricts federal takings, it does not place such limitations on state and local governments. Some states, such as New Jersey, do have some limits on the use of eminent domain built into their state constitutions to protect property takings from benefitting individuals, developers, or corporations.[6] Other states do not.

Controversies surrounding the use of eminent domain continue. Current examples include the taking or threat of taking private property for the construction of the Keystone XL and other pipelines,[7] the threat of taking private property to construct protective sand dunes along the beachfront areas of New Jersey that were devastated by Hurricane Sandy,[8] and cities attempting to halt massive foreclosures by using eminent domain to condemn underwater-mortgaged properties, buy them at market value, and refinance them at lower rates so that large numbers of families are not displaced.[9] Whether these efforts will succeed depends upon pending court decisions.

Zoning

Zoning is a statutory planning tool that allows municipalities to control local land uses in delineated areas of a master or regional plan. Rapid urbanization caused U.S. cities to expand both outward and upward after 1850. Their uncontrolled growth became a challenge for anyone working or residing in, or traveling through, American cities. Poor neighborhoods lost sunlight and air from both the increasing numbers and heights of tenement buildings (see Chapter 1). Encroaching warehouses with their shipping and transport traffic, factories with their belching smokestacks, slaughterhouses with their noises and smells, and other nuisance land uses assaulted urban quality of life. It was obvious to all that the situation was worsening by the year.

By 1920, more than half of all Americans lived in cities and, with the trend toward increasing urbanization showing no signs of abating, something needed to be done. The stars aligned for three events to solidify zoning as a standard urban planning practice during the 1920s. The first two events were the publication of "standard acts" or model legislation that states could use to develop their own zoning and planning statutes. The third event was a landmark U.S. Supreme Court decision.

Stuart Meck, former national president of the APA, tells the story of how the two standard acts came about.[10] The story begins at the 1913 National Conference on City Planning in Chicago, Illinois. Proceedings from that conference contain several model acts, including ones on eminent domain, creating city planning departments, and regulating plans (zoning) for lots. Before the end of the decade, 10 states had authorized some of their cities to enact zoning to regulate patterns of urban growth, but these regulations were not standardized.

In 1920, President Warren G. Harding appointed Herbert Hoover Secretary of Commerce, a position he continued to hold under President Calvin Coolidge. Upon taking the position, Hoover's interests in housing and city planning quickly became apparent. He appointed a committee, the Advisory Committee on Zoning (later the Advisory Committee on City Planning and Zoning), and tasked it with drafting model statutes or "standard acts" that the states could readily adopt as their own. The committee released the Standard State Zoning Enabling Act (SZEA) in 1924, with revisions in 1926.[11] The SZEA model act grants zoning power to cities and incorporated villages to regulate and restrict

- The height, number of stories, and size of buildings and other structures
- The percentage of a lot that can be occupied (including size of yards, courts, and other open spaces)
- The density of population
- The location and use of land for trade, industry, resident, or other purposes

The SZEA also calls for the boundaries of zoning districts to be recommended by a zoning commission and for regulations and restrictions to be administered "in accordance with a comprehensive plan." Many states adopted the SZEA, noting that such regulations not only improved quality of life in cities and lessened land use conflicts, but they also aided in preserving property values. Some states, such as New York, do not require that the comprehensive plan be encased in a single document; it can grow organically.[12] Other states, such as California, are highly prescriptive about what must be in a comprehensive plan.[13]

The second model act was the Standard City Planning Enabling Act (SCPEA) of 1928, intended to complement the SZEA.[14] Six subjects are covered in this model act:

1. Organization and power of a planning commission to prepare and adopt a master plan
2. Content of the master plan
3. Adoption of a master street plan (by the governing body)
4. Approval of all public improvements (by the planning commission)
5. Control of private subdivisions of land
6. Establishment of a regional planning commission and regional plan

The change in terminology from "comprehensive plan" to "master plan" between the two standard acts and their adoption by various states has led to some confusion about the use of the terms. Some planning textbooks suggest that municipalities adopt comprehensive plans whereas special districts adopt master plans, but this is not always the case. Some states use one term or the other exclusively in their statutes, thus restricting the municipalities in that state to using a single term. Regardless of the term used, the model act includes information on zoning restrictions within the area of administration.

The third event solidifying zoning as a planning tool was *Euclid v. Ambler*,[15] a 1926 U.S. Supreme Court decision that pitted the village of Euclid, Ohio, against Ambler Realty. Euclid, a suburb of Cleveland, passed zoning regulations that prohibited Ambler from developing its land holdings for industrial use. The court found that Euclid had a valid interest in regulating the land uses within its jurisdiction, a ruling that has not since been challenged. As a result, Euclidian zoning rapidly became a powerful planning tool. It allows for dividing a municipality into land use districts (residential, commercial, industrial, and other) and limiting the activities that can occur within each zone.

Euclidian zoning is effective for regulating density and land use; however, many planners consider the tool both inflexible and outdated. It is inflexible, as any alternative to existing zoning regulations requires that a variance be obtained after a discretionary review by a zoning board. It is outdated, as the land use problems of the previous century have changed. The belching smokestacks are now only remnants of the past; dealing with urban sprawl requires increasing urban density rather than dispersing it; and reducing commuting times requires bringing commercial and industrial areas closer to residential ones.

One alternative to Euclidian zoning is performance zoning. Performance zoning attempts to retain the character of communities and protect their natural resources rather than restricting particular types of land use to designated areas. It does this through three performance criteria: minimum open space, maximum density, and maximum impervious surface. An example of performance zoning comes from the Bucks County Planning Commission in Pennsylvania.[16] Passed in 1973, the performance zoning codes require a developer to first identify the natural resources on a site (wetlands, floodplains, and steep slopes, in particular) and then determine the size of the buildable area that will still protect these resources. Any type of development is then permitted as long as it meets the open space minimum and does not exceed the maximum density for the district.

Some planners hailed performance zoning as an excellent response to the rigid nature of Euclidian zoning. Specifically, it required fewer administrative actions (variances, appeals, and requirements for re-zoning were eliminated) and allowed for a range of land uses as long as the developer protected natural resources.[17] The downside of performance zoning is that it is not designed to create places where people want to live, places that provide them with ready access to shopping, services, and jobs. (See Chapter 10 for more about zoning and building codes.)

Planned Unit Developments

An alternative to Euclidian and performance zoning is the planned unit development (PUD), a special district that may range from a simple residential cluster to a large master-planned community with mixed uses. PUDs can be efficient designs for preserving open space. They serve the interests of both developers and municipalities by providing lower costs for street and utility construction and maintenance.[18]

Consider that a developer applies to a municipality for approval of a PUD that includes housing and office space, retail space, or both. If approved, the PUD becomes a floating zone, or a district superimposed on the master plan that has its own land use regulations. Homeowners associations (HOAs) often manage residential PUDs, providing amenities such as a community pool or recreational facility, as well as the maintenance of common areas. The HOA may place restrictive covenants (deed restrictions) on what homeowners may do with their property. The covenants may restrict the height and types of landscaping, or the type and color of building materials.

The commercial ventures in a PUD may have deed restrictions on the types of services allowed, or the types and amount of signage and lighting permitted. The goal of these restrictions is to impose conformity on the aesthetics of the overall community—the visual experience of anyone traversing the PUD. When PUDs are used for "infill" (filling in gaps in already developed areas) where zoning already exists, it can become a challenge to craft sophisticated legislation to create and manage the new development project.[19]

When zoning regulations and restrictive covenants come into conflict, the more restrictive of the two is likely to be upheld in court. For instance, a city may zone an area for commercial use with 10-foot setbacks, but deed restrictions on properties in that zone may limit their use to residences with 25-foot setbacks. In cases such as these, the stricter limits are likely to prevail.

Consider that an owner may donate a property to a municipality but it has a restrictive covenant that limits the use of the property to open-space purposes such as parks and recreational fields. Unless otherwise stated, this limitation on use of the property holds into perpetuity ("goes with the land"). If the municipality accepts the property, it may never be used for a new school, library, hospital, or other needed facility, nor can it be sold to another owner for any purpose other than open space. Some restrictive covenants prevent hunting or trapping into perpetuity, preventing communities from culling diseased animals (such as wasting deer), or even removing threatening ones such as overpopulations of bears. Some deed restrictions prevent the removal of trees, even if they threaten to damage neighboring structures or pose fire threats. Municipalities must think long and hard before accepting properties, even free ones, with restrictive covenants that last into perpetuity.

Perhaps the most damning use of restrictive covenants has been to prevent select racial and ethnic groups from purchasing properties in neighborhoods or even in entire cities. In 1917, a U.S. Supreme Court decision in *Buchanan v. Warley* found that the racial zoning ordinance of Louisville, Kentucky, violated the 14th Amendment's due protection clause.[20] Although that decision addressed the unconstitutionality of racially restrictive zoning practices, it did not address private contracts. As a result, racially based restrictive covenants on property transfers became common as a means to prevent blacks, Jews, Catholics, Chinese, Greeks, Japanese, and other groups from integrating neighborhoods.

The U.S. Commission on Civil Rights notes that exclusionary covenants became so common that by 1940 more than 80 percent of the properties in Chicago, Illinois, and Los Angeles, California, prevented blacks from purchasing them.[21] Racially based restrictive covenants on property deeds across the nation persisted until the 1948 U.S. Supreme Court *Shelley v. Kraemer* decision determined that they were unconstitutional.[22] Although such restrictions are no longer enforceable, they remain in many property deeds, testimony to the nation's racially biased history.

Downzoning

In contrast to increasing residential density by using PUDs or cluster housing, administrative units may attempt to reduce density or restrict urban sprawl through downzoning. Downzoning in urban areas may happen when an area is cleared, such as when an apartment building is demolished and replaced with single-family townhomes, or when an abandoned industrial complex is replaced with a smaller footprint of retail shops. It may also happen when an urbanizing area wants to prevent real estate speculation, to shift density toward select sections of a city (such as near a transit stop), or as a first step toward historic preservation.

An example of urban downzoning comes from New York City where, during the late 1990s, the public became frustrated by high-rise apartment towers sprouting up in traditional brownstone neighborhoods. Local residents were also frustrated by the bulldozing of small wood-frame houses in the outer boroughs to make space for McMansions. Writing for *Politico*, Sarah Laskow states that a "downzoning uprising" swept across all five boroughs.[23] At the same time, however, New York City's population was bursting at the seams, and the need for additional housing was irrefutable. The Bloomberg administration responded by rezoning 120 areas of the city, a massive effort that included downzoning to preserve the character of select neighborhoods:

> In 2010, N.Y.U.'s Furman Center for Real Estate and Urban Policy found that, of the 188,000 lots that had been rezoned between 2003 and 2007, 14 percent had been upzoned, 23 percent downzoned, and 63 percent had not had their development capacity changed by more than 10 percent.[23]

Places such as Ozone Park, Queens, were downzoned so that some commercial infill was permitted along select streets, but residential development was restricted to low-rise and single-family structures.[24] As many New York City neighborhoods did not benefit from downzoning, their community organizations circulated a petition calling for an end "to the violence that real estate developers have inflicted on our skyline, parks, public areas, and cityscape with the proliferation of dramatically over-scaled buildings."[25]

Downzoning in rural areas occurs when limitations are imposed on development by requiring large lot sizes or restricting changes in land use. For instance, a farmer may be prevented from selling his property to a developer, even if farming is no longer economically feasible in the area, or if personal factors prevent the farmer from continuing in that occupation. When a farmer is prevented from benefitting from the worth of his property (equivalent to a "taking"), the natural place for him to go to seek redress is in the courts.[26] This poses a conundrum for communities as preserving farmland is considered one aspect of communities practicing "smart growth" (development and conservation strategies that protect human health and the natural environment).[27]

An example of downzoning to protect the rural nature of an area and its natural resources is that of Baltimore County, Maryland. Beginning in 1975, Baltimore County downzoned rural areas from one dwelling per acre to one dwelling per five acres. Farmlands surrounding the reservoirs that provide drinking water to the Baltimore area were designated one dwelling to 50-acre zoning. As a result, 90 percent of the county's population lived on 30 percent of the county's land in 2000, and little land was left for development. While the rural nature of much of the county has been maintained, farmland in the county has decreased because five-acre-zoned lots are insufficient for farming.[28]

Form-Based Codes

As an alternative to zoning practices, some urban communities adopted form-based codes (FBCs)—regulations that shape the physical form of their neighborhoods. The theory behind why FBCs should work can be traced to what is now considered a classic book about urban form written by Jane Jacobs in 1961—*The Death and Life of American Cities.*[29] Simply put, vibrant cities require human interactions, with connected sidewalks that allow large numbers of people to go about their daily lives and act as social controls. Jacobs notes that the key to creating bustling streets that hold the interest of pedestrians, and neighborhoods where people want to be, is mixed use. FBCs encourage mixed uses (a combination of residential with commercial, cultural, institutional, or industrial land uses) in an effort to generate lively communities with a great deal of social interaction.

In contrast to Euclidian zoning, which restricts land use within districts, FBCs divide a community into neighborhoods and street corridors designed to have a consistent character. The codes consider how buildings relate to the streetscape so that they encourage pedestrian activity, provide attractive public spaces, and allow a variety of mixed uses. Much of the literature on FBCs, however, warns that too much detail in the codes is likely to create implementation problems. This means that FBCs can become as inflexible as Euclidian zoning (requiring a burdensome number of applications for zoning variances) or PUDs (requiring an inordinate number of applications for HOA board approvals). Readers seeking to improve the social interactions of their communities through planning practices will find the Chicago Metropolitan Planning Agency's comprehensive handbook on implementing FBCs helpful.[30]

Special Districts

Some open land or built areas may require unique forms of protection, and they may be designated as historic or environmentally sensitive districts with special regulations. For instance, the U.S. Department of the Interior, National Park Service, designates national historic sites and places them on the National Register of Historic Places. Individuals may apply to place their properties on the register, and this will not restrict their use or disposition of their property, although it may provide access to some benefits.[31]

States and localities may also have their own historic designations. The first historic district designation in the United States was the Old and Historic District created by city ordinance in Charleston, South Carolina, in 1931. The French Quarter was designated by the City of New Orleans as a historic district in 1937, and the Beacon Hill Historic District of Boston was so designated in 1955.[32] Cities may also use historic designations to maintain the character of select buildings and districts, placing restrictions on their use. For example, Grand Central Terminal was designated a New York City Landmark in

1967 and placed on the National Register of Historic places in 1976. Penn Central owned the property and applied to the New York City Landmarks Preservation Commission for approval to construct a 50-story building above the landmark. When the application was denied, Penn Central sued, claiming the denial was equivalent to the use of eminent domain and the company's loss of property rights should be justly compensated. In 1978, the U.S. Supreme Court decided the *Penn Central Transportation Co. v. City of New York* case, finding that the original use of the property was for rail transit and the building could continue to be used in the same way. Thus, there was no taking and Penn Central was not entitled to compensation.

Environmentally sensitive districts, such as floodplains, hillsides prone to rock or mudslides, or limited groundwater resources may require specific types of restrictions or zoning ordinances. An example of ordinances designed to protect groundwater resources comes from Austin, Texas. Much of that city sits above an environmentally sensitive aquifer that supplies drinking water to more than 50,000 people, as well as supplying water for the Colorado River. To protect the aquifer, the Austin Water Protection Department has a "Grow Green" program that promotes

- Sustainable landscaping to reduce watering
- An integrated pest management practices to encourage less use of toxic chemicals that may enter the water supply
- A "Scoop the Poop" program to reduce pet waste and prevent health and water quality problems
- A series of watershed ordinances to limit the amount of impervious surfaces and control stormwater runoff[33]

Land use controls are used for a wide variety of purposes, including protecting natural and man-made resources, encouraging more habitable and functional cities, and planning for future controlled growth. A lack of land use controls may lead to unfettered growth, resulting in a degraded quality of life with snarled traffic and intolerable living conditions. The opposite is also true, however, as too many land use controls may strangle economic development and lead to a stifled or degraded quality of life with little promise for improvement. The goal for planning, then, is to create and implement land use controls in a balanced fashion, so that they serve to improve living and economic conditions that benefit both a community's residential and economic interests.

Economic Development

Economic development is an integral part of a comprehensive plan. The goal of economic development is to create and maintain desirable jobs that provide a good standard of living. When personal income and wealth are increased, the local tax base increases.

As a result, better community services are demanded and provided, and the general livability of the community is improved.

Expenditures on economic development are investments that help shape the future of a community according to its own values. The planner's role is to evaluate plans for community development and to propose those that are feasible for public consideration. Before they can do that, planners must first understand how their local economy works in relation to the larger region in which it sits. Performing an economic base analysis, a technique that calculates total economic activity as the sum of two categories—basic activities that bring in wealth from outside the region, and non-basic activities that service the region—does this. Without income from basic (export) activities, non-basic (local) activities wither.

An economic base analysis begins with the analyst classifying activities by sector. The sectors for basic activities are agriculture, forestry, mining, manufacturing, state and local government, and tourism. Those for non-basic activities are local government, retail, schools, construction, and utilities. Information about the activity in each sector is estimated from wage and employment data, usually obtained from the state. Interviews with and information from major employers (the regional economic base) further inform the analysis by estimating trends in sales, expectations for increasing or decreasing the number of employees, any changing needs for land use and space, and more. The results of the economic base analysis aid the planner in understanding how larger economic forces might have an impact on local decisions made by the community.

Once the larger economic forces are understood, planners undertake a market study of their local economy. The market study contains information about local demographics and provides an inventory of all existing land uses and built space. The planner then evaluates potential economic opportunities for his locale and identifies any existing regional competition. They must identify whether a project is feasible by identifying barriers (such as zoning or other regulations) and whether existing infrastructure and the local political climate will support the project. For example, is there community resistance to certain types of growth? Is there community support for providing incentives such as tax abatements or other subsidies to entice certain types of projects?

If the market study supports proposing projects that will advance economic development, the planner must then enter the arena of economic recruitment. Recruited projects should be assessed for environmental, health, social, and economic impacts. Developers generate a pro-forma analysis (a projection of the financial return on an investment) to determine whether they should or should not go forward with a particular project. If the bottom line of the pro-forma is that the project will not be profitable, the developer may demand concessions such as tax abatements, public–private partnerships for large-scale projects, or other types of subsidies in order to realize a profit on the endeavor. It is incumbent upon the planner to evaluate the developer's statements carefully and to report to municipal officials whether concessions in subsidies, zoning regulations, and the increased load on infrastructure will result in a net increase in jobs, tax revenues, or a reduction of local debt. If the answer is yes, and if the project is acceptable to the community, it may move into the implementation phase.

Economic development projects may take many forms, depending on the vision the community has for its own future and its willingness to be proactive in adapting to structural changes in the economy. For instance, what are the physical and human assets the community has to offer? Does it have a skilled workforce, access to transportation nodes, or environmental resources that make it attractive? Does the political leadership foster a good business climate? Does it take regional collaborations seriously? Is there a willingness to invest in innovation? The decisions community leaders make about economic development projects will depend on the answers to these questions and many more.

Examples of economic development projects include attracting new residents by creating PUDs for retirees, transit villages for commuters, or residential units targeting select demographic groups, such as millennials. Some communities seek economic development through tourism by providing improved access to historic districts or by developing new cultural centers or theater and arts districts. If creating jobs is the primary concern, projects may focus on retail or industry, parks and recreation, or the provision of flexible office space. The decisions made about local economic development require cooperation between those proposing development projects and the local governmental structure, hopefully guided by good planning practices and community support. These practices should be balanced, as dependence on one type of economic development may leave a community vulnerable if that sector decides to leave.

The need for a balanced economic approach to planning cannot be overstated. Consider that if an existing industry providing the majority of jobs in a community decides it will relocate to become more competitive, the dependent community will lose its entire economic base. For example, the cities of the Rust Belt (those located in the Northeast and Midwestern sections of the United States) suffered significantly under the processes of globalization and deindustrialization over the past decades. Planners developed strategies to rebuild the tax base and revenue streams of their cities based on the physical and human assets of their jurisdictions. Some of the plans called for the creation of microbrewery, artisanal, or cultural districts to draw a young and "creative" class into their economies. Others recommended tax incentives for "green industries" and the removal of crumbling buildings, to be replaced with parks and waterfront districts. A boon to some areas was the availability of a reliable and fairly inexpensive energy—natural gas—as well as access to transportation nodes and a supportive political culture willing to guarantee the infrastructure and other needs for new ventures to survive.

Some of these balanced economic development efforts were successful in bringing businesses back to formerly Rust Belt cities. As examples, Google, Apple, Bosch, Disney, IBM, Intel, and Uber have expanded their footprint in Pittsburgh, Pennsylvania, because of the relative cost advantage to expanding there rather than along the coasts. Cleveland, Ohio, installed the nation's first 100-gigabit fiber optic network and developed a health-tech corridor that has drawn more than $1 billion in venture capital. Its Rock & Roll Hall of Fame also stands as a significant tourist draw. Young, well-educated workers (particularly engineers) are locating to these and other reviving Rust Belt cities because of low housing costs and high-paying job opportunities. The cities' new businesses and residents add to their tax base each year, generating a true comeback from the economic disaster brought about by their former reliance on sole industries that abandoned them.[34] These cities stand out as excellent examples of planned, balanced economic development strategies.

Housing and Community Development

After World War II, developers responded to the demand for housing by building new homes in undeveloped areas near cities rather than redeveloping areas within urban centers. As middle-class families moved to the ever-expanding suburbs, minorities and the poor remained behind with declining urban housing stock and reduced public services. The zoning practices of the previous half century, along with changes in industrial production, left large parcels of urban land with derelict buildings or empty city lots that may or may not have been contaminated with toxic chemicals. These deserted areas attracted criminal activity and served as depressingly visual reminders of urban economic decline. Greenberg, Popper, and West named these pockmarked areas of obvious decline Temporarily Obsolete Abandoned Derelict Sites (TOADS).[35]

To many, particularly young families, suburbia seemed to be the appropriate escape from declining urban environments. The reality, however, was that the rapid rise of suburban communities required an enormous amount of new infrastructure and services (e.g., roads and schools; police, fire, and emergency medical services), and these were costly for the new communities to provide. Property taxes increased, commuting time became onerous, and children required buses to transport them to new regional schools. Suburban families quickly discovered they were isolated without one or more automobiles—vehicles that not only took the breadwinner to work but that also could transport family members for health care, shopping, and other services. Indeed, those who fled the cities had their everyday lives impacted by urban sprawl, defined by Ewing and colleagues as

- Dispersed low-density development
- Rigidly separated homes, shops, and workplaces
- A network of roads marked by huge blocks and poor access
- A lack of well-defined, thriving activity centers, such as downtowns and town centers[36]

By the 1990s, planners were struggling contemporaneously with the decline of urban centers and urban sprawl. Two movements sprang up to address these issues at about this time, the New Urbanism and Smart Growth. Although the movements served different constituencies and different purposes, most planners found their philosophies useful for addressing specific needs.

The New Urbanism

The isolation of the suburbs caused by automobile dependency, the explanations offered by Jane Jacobs and others about places where people want to be, and the contrasts between declining American cities and "livable" cities in Europe led to a rethinking of urban form. In 1993, architects, designers, engineers, planners, and citizens with urban interests were brought together under the umbrella of a new Chicago-based organization, the Congress for the New Urbanism (CNU). The CNU meets annually in various U.S. cities, hosting participants from around the globe to discuss issues of the New Urbanism. The organization notes that New Urbanists want to return to "human-scale" neighborhoods by using zoning and design reform. The CNU claims:

> New Urbanists have been responsible for creating and popularizing many now-common development patterns and strategies, including mixed-use development, transit-oriented development, traditional neighborhood design, integrating design standards into affordable housing, and designing complete and beautiful streets.[37]

The principles of the New Urbanism have been applied to the creation of entire communities called "New Urbanist Towns," as well as to sections of municipalities designated as walkable neighborhoods or transit-oriented development. While many New Urbanist design efforts have been successful in creating places where people want to be, others have not. An example that was not a resounding success was the Disney creation of an ideal master-planned community—Celebration, Florida. Celebration has a town center, a variety of housing stock, and markets itself as a walkable community for a population of about 8,000 persons. Whereas some new residents found the community ideal for their needs, others complained that it was lacking in diversity and was so perfect it was just plain "creepy."[38] Despite the occasionally less-than-stellar outcome, the New Urbanism has been successful in pushing for pedestrian-based, socially diverse neighborhoods with a built environment (see Chapter 9 on the creation of Stapleton, Colorado) that should eventually lead to the creation of sustainable cities (those that meet present needs without compromising the city's future).

Smart Growth

The second movement born in the 1990s was Smart Growth, defined as "development that is compact, contiguous to existing urban areas, well connected by a grid-like network of through-streets, characterized by a diverse mix of land uses, and relatively dense."[39] The Smart Growth movement came about as multiple public and private organizations began encouraging the updating of land use controls to emphasize compact development rather than sprawl. This may be best exemplified by the APA's launch of a seven-year project entitled Growing Smart in 1994. The Growing Smart project culminated in a legislative guidebook with model statutes designed to replace the zoning and planning ones drafted in the 1920s (see the SZEA and SCPEA in "Zoning," earlier in this chapter).[40]

Of particular interest is that the APA guidebook offers as model legislation the Smart Growth Act passed by Maryland in 1997. That act prohibits state funding for projects unless they meet select guidelines (minimum density requirements and adequate plans for water and sewer systems). It encourages the redevelopment of brownfields (properties contaminated or potentially contaminated with a hazardous substance) and grayfields (outdated properties, such as abandoned shopping malls, which do not require extensive environmental remediation) by offering developers legal incentives (limited liability) and financial ones such as grants, low-interest loans, and tax credits. The model act allows for investment in central cities, distressed areas that require investment (sometimes called enterprise zones), and other areas targeted for redevelopment by various planning agencies.

While the APA project was ongoing, the Natural Resources Defense Council and the Surface Transportation Policy Project jointly developed a "Smart Growth toolkit" to assist local and state governments in producing walkable neighborhoods and transit-oriented development, crossover interests of the New Urbanism.[41] At about the same time, the U.S. Environmental Protection Agency (EPA) joined with various nonprofit and government agencies to create the Smart Growth Network of more than 40 organizations. Numerous academic and trade journals began to publish articles on the economic, environmental, and human health costs of sprawl. A diffuse agenda for the Smart Growth movement began to develop—agendas as varied as those of commuters, developers, environmentalists, farmers, and public health advocates. Each group took up the mantle of Smart Growth, creating its own Smart Growth toolkit. It should not surprise anyone to learn that a Smart Growth toolkit for realtors includes creating options for housing[42] or that one of the important Smart Growth tools of the Association of State and Territorial Health Officials is improving access to health care.[43]

The variation in Smart Growth toolkits (providing something for everyone) speaks to the lack of a core to the Smart Growth movement. Indeed, Smart Growth now includes promoting local food enterprises and downtown revitalization, improving transportation and traffic management, maintaining infrastructure, preparing for and recovering from natural disasters (resiliency), and generally creating healthy and sustainable communities. The EPA notes that expansion of the Smart Growth movement is a strength in that it will "help protect our health and natural environment(s) and make out communities more attractive, economically stronger, and more socially diverse."[44]

Improving the Food Supply

The United States has highly advanced food distribution and retail systems that allow those with means to obtain fresh meat and dairy products, as well as out-of-season fresh fruits and vegetables from around the globe on a year-round basis. Supermarkets, the unparalleled supplier of these foodstuffs, are likely to locate in suburban communities where land is available for large buildings with many aisles of shelf space and where shoppers can park so they can take home cartloads of items. By contrast, bodegas, convenience stores, corner grocers, or food kiosks that stock mostly processed foods with longer shelf lives serve residents of urban neighborhoods. This lack of accessibility to fresh produce and healthy foods plays an important role in perpetuating food insecurity and poor nutrition, particularly among low-income households.

The U.S. Department of Agriculture (USDA) notes that food insecurity and poor nutrition are not only problems for individuals with low incomes but are also community-wide problems created by the distance to a store, a limited number of stores in an area, and lack of access to transportation.[45] Thus, community food security should be within the purview of urban planning, yet it has been largely absent from the planning literature, from local plans developed by professional planners, and from urban planning classrooms.[45] Indeed, surveys of urban planning agencies across the United States found little to no involvement of municipal planning agencies in the food system.[46–48]

In 2002, the USDA published a Community Food Assessment Toolkit to help municipalities determine whether their food supply is safe, culturally acceptable, nutritionally adequate, and sustainable.[49] The toolkit has six assessment components:

1. A profile of community socioeconomic and demographic characteristics: income levels, number of persons in poverty
2. A profile of community food resources: number of food stores, kiosks, and open-air food markets
3. Assessment of household food security: number of persons served by food pantries, local food assistance programs
4. Assessment of food resource accessibility: barriers to food shopping, hours of food assistance programs
5. Assessment of food availability and affordability: food selection and pricing
6. Assessment of community food production resources: loss of farmland, availability of locally grown food and community gardens

Some of the terms used to describe issues related to community food resources, particularly in impoverished areas, are food deserts and food swamps. Food deserts are communities with no access to fresh fruits and vegetables due to a lack of supermarkets or large grocery stores, farmers' markets, or other healthy food providers. A food swamp is a neighborhood where unhealthy foods are more readily available than healthy ones, such as a number of fast food restaurants but no large grocery store.[50] Both food deserts and food swamps have been designated as important to rectify by the UDSA as part of First Lady Michelle Obama's efforts to reduce obesity in the United States. Planners are increasingly aware of the need to provide healthy food opportunities as part of local development plans (see Chapter 7 case study).

Improving Transportation and Traffic Management

Planners are aware of the need to balance auto dependency in urban areas with heavy and light rail, buses, bicycles, and walking. Planners must consider not only the needs of commuters getting to and from work as quickly as possible but also the needs of children, the elderly, and the disabled. To illustrate the importance of considering these populations, we point out that the four most dangerous urban areas for pedestrians in the United States are in resort and retirement areas in Florida: (1) Orlando–Kissimmee, (2) Tampa–St. Petersburg–Clearwater, (3) Jacksonville, and (4) Miami–Fort Lauderdale–Pompano Beach.[51]

Traffic calming tools such as speed bumps, one-way streets, traffic lights, timed crossings, sidewalks with grass buffer strips, and curb ramps provide some protection for pedestrians. Unfortunately, reducing auto traffic in built-up areas remains a planning and public health challenge (see Chapter 5 case study). Planners have embraced transit-oriented development (TOD)—housing clustered around public transit stops—in an effort to increase density and reduce commuter auto traffic (Figure 2.2). The results, however, have been mixed. For instance, TODs in Jersey City, New Jersey, did lure new residents who had been commuting to New York City from the suburbs. However, many of them simply brought their autos with them rather than surrender to sole reliance on public transit. Similar issues have plagued cities such as Chicago.[53]

Many cities have resorted to requiring residents to purchase parking permits to discourage local auto ownership as well as parking by day trippers. Others have restricted parking in downtown areas to underground or vertical lots, and significantly raised parking costs in both metered and public lots to discourage auto use (New York City; Honolulu, Hawaii; and Boston, Massachusetts, in particular). To further discourage auto use and to encourage more walking and biking, some cities have designated select streets as pedestrian walkways and added protective barriers to create safe bike lanes. More than 70 U.S. cities have instituted bike-sharing programs, as have several major universities.[54]

Will America's love of the automobile continue? Some are beginning to question whether it will. After the recession of 2008, the number of vehicles on American roads declined.[55] Millennials have already found that Zipcars serve them well in urban areas. Many now choose to carpool, use Uber, or take public transit where they can continue to work (and text) while others take the responsibility for getting them where they want to

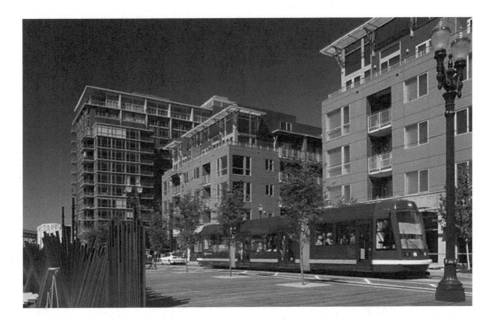

Source: Reprinted from Smart Growth Tulsa.[52]

Figure 2.2. Transit-Oriented Development in Tulsa, Oklahoma

go. Planners use such information to persuade additional drivers to change their travel habits and to convince city administrators to work toward integrated transportation systems that are healthier for all.

Infrastructure, Sustainability, and Resilience

Maintaining roads and bridges, as well as communication and electricity lines, is essential to the American way of life. Potholes that go unfilled or bridge struts that rust out can be devastating to both commerce and human health. Societies need to safeguard their potable water supplies, as well as their pipelines, ports, and other interchange locations. Indeed, without sufficient and reliable infrastructure, cities and regions can come to a halt. To address infrastructure needs, planners may be called upon to redesign traffic patterns, improve energy and water efficiency, or develop waste reduction/recycling plans. All of these services and more are needed for continued and sustainable growth.

Keeping communities functioning may be business as usual, but doing it with an eye to a sustainable future is laudable. Both the New Urbanism and Smart Growth movements encourage the use of green building techniques, defined as "the planning, design, construction, and operations of buildings [that addresses] energy use, water use, indoor environmental quality, material [selection], and the building's effects on its site."[56]

Green building is a concept promoted in 1994 by the U.S. Green Building Council, and it encourages architects, engineers, planners, and other professionals to become certified in Leadership in Energy and Environmental Design (LEED). LEED certification can be achieved at four levels (certified, silver, gold, or platinum) based on the number of points accrued. Green buildings have lower costs to operate and are preferred by many businesses seeking to relocate or upgrade their facilities (see Chapter 10). Furthermore, Fannie Mae announced in 2015 that it would provide lower interest rates for LEED-certified multifamily properties.[57]

Akin to sustainability is the concept of resilience, the ability of a system to adapt to or recover from a shock or disturbance. Concerns about global climate change (rising sea levels, droughts), as well as recovery after human-induced disasters (such as the 9/11 attacks) and naturally induced ones (such as Hurricane Katrina in 2005) pushed some cities and regions to develop plans for efficient evacuation routes, access to emergency care, and redundant communications networks. For others, resilience meant improving infrastructure to draw new commercial ventures in order to ensure economic survival in a global economy.

After Hurricane Sandy in the fall of 2011, U.S. federal agencies began developing Infrastructure Resilience Guidelines to deal with prioritizing funding efforts related to human and natural disaster recovery.[58] Linked to federal funding, resilience became a priority for city managers, nongovernmental organizations, politicians, and certainly urban planners. As it had with Smart Growth, the literature on resilience exploded. Dozens of books and innumerable journal articles on planning for resilience became available between 2012 and 2015. As with Smart Growth, toolkits and workbooks became available for communities to use to plan for and measure their resilience.[59] The U.S. Department of Commerce put out a Community Resilience Planning Guide in 2015,[60] as well as guidance for economic resilience in 2016.[61] It appears that resilience is going to be with the planning community for the foreseeable future (see Chapter 6 case studies).

Professional Ethics

In 1992, the APA set out ethical guidelines for planners, recognizing that issues facing communities often involve stakeholders with conflicting values. Despite the fact that there is likely to be conflict in the planning process, the APA guidelines call on planners to

1. Recognize the rights of citizens to participate in planning decisions.
2. Strive to give citizens (including those who lack formal organization or influence) full, clear, and accurate information on planning issues and the opportunity to have a meaningful role in the development of plans and programs.
3. Strive to expand choice and opportunity for all persons, recognizing a special responsibility to plan for the needs of disadvantaged groups and persons.

4. Assist in the clarification of community goals, objectives, and policies in plan making.

5. Ensure that reports, records, and any other nonconfidential information that is, or will be, available to decision-makers is made available to the public in a convenient format and sufficiently in advance of any decision.

6. Strive to protect the integrity of the natural environment and the heritage of the built environment.

7. Pay special attention to the interrelatedness of decisions and the long-range consequences of present actions.[62]

These APA professional guidelines may be written for planners, but the statements could just as easily be applied to public health professionals. Indeed, planners use the same population-based data sets, public survey results, statistical software packages, and other tools designed for working with communities, as do public health professionals. Chapter 3 covers the building blocks of public health, and Part II of this book contains descriptions of the tools used by both professions, along with case studies to describe the use of the tools in the real world.

References

1. Sutherland J. What is city planning? Available at: https://www.planning.org/kidsandcommunity/whatisplanning. Accessed March 2, 2017.

2. Library of Congress via Wikimedia Commons. Plan of the City of Washington, March 1792, by Andrew Ellicott, revised from Pierre Charles L'Enfant; Thackara & Vallance, Philadelphia 1792. Available at: https://commons.wikimedia.org/wiki/File:L'Enfant_plan.jpg. Accessed March 22, 2017.

3. US Department of Justice, Environment and Natural Resources Division. History of the federal use of eminent domain. 2015. Available at: https://www.justice.gov/enrd/history-federal-use-eminent-domain. Accessed March 22, 2016.

4. *Kelo v New London*, 545 US 469 (2005).

5. Bush GW. Executive Order: Protecting the property rights of the American people. The White House. 2006. Available at: http://georgewbush-whitehouse.archives.gov/news/releases/2006/06/20060623-10.html. Accessed January 31, 2016.

6. New Jersey State Constitution, Article 8, Section 3. Available at: http://www.njleg.state.nj.us/lawsconstitution/constitution.asp. Accessed May 6, 2016.

7. Israel J, Valentine K. TransCanada is seizing people's land to build Keystone, but conservatives have been dead silent. ClimateProgress. 2015. Available at: http://thinkprogress.org/climate/2015/03/01/3625804/keystone-kelo-eminent-domain-property. Accessed March 22, 2016.

8. Spoto M. Eminent domain will help expand public space at beaches, state says for 1st time. 2016. Available at: http://www.nj.com/ocean/index.ssf/2016/02/eminent_domain_will_help_expand_public_space_at_be.html. Accessed March 22, 2016.

9. Hockett R. Paying Paul and robbing no one: an eminent domain solution for underwater mortgage debt. *Curr Issues Econ Financ.* 2013;13(5):109.

10. Meck S. Model planning and zoning legislation: a short history. In: *Modernizing State Planning Statutes: The Growing Smart Working Papers.* Vol 1. Chicago, IL: American Planning Association Planning Advisory Service; 1996.

11. A Standard State Zoning Enabling Act. Washington, DC: US Department of Commerce, Advisory Committee on City Planning and Zoning; 1926.

12. State of New York, Division of Local Government Services. Zoning and the comprehensive plan. 2015. Available at: https://www.dos.ny.gov/lg/publications/Zoning_and_the_Comprehensive_Plan.pdf. Accessed February 2, 2016.

13. Governor's Office of Planning and Research. General plan guidelines. 2003. Available at: https://www.opr.ca.gov/docs/General_Plan_Guidelines_2003.pdf. Accessed February 2, 2016.

14. US Department of Commerce, Advisory Committee on City Planning and Zoning. A Standard City Planning Enabling Act. 1928. Available at: https://planning-org-uploaded-media.s3.amazonaws.com/legacy_resources/growingsmart/pdf/CPEnabling%20Act1928.pdf. Accessed March 2, 2017.

15. US Supreme Court. *Village of Euclid v Ambler Realty Co.* (1926). Available at: https://supreme.justia.com/cases/federal/us/272/365/case.html. Accessed January 24, 2016.

16. Performance zoning model ordinance. Doylestown, PA: Bucks County Planning Commission; 1996.

17. Kendig L. *Performance Zoning: Lane Kendig.* Chicago, IL: Planners Press, American Planning Association; 1980.

18. Burchell R, Hughes J. *Planned Unit Development: New Communities American Style.* New Brunswick, NJ: Center for Urban Policy Research, Rutgers University; 1973.

19. Mandelker DR. Legislation for planned unit developments and master-planned communities. *The Urban Lawyer.* 2008;40(3):419–449.

20. *Buchanan v Warley,* 245 US 60 (1917). Available at: https://supreme.justia.com/cases/federal/us/245/60/case.html. Accessed May 6, 2016.

21. US Commission on Civil Rights. Understanding fair housing. Clearinghouse Publication 42. 1973. Available at: http://www.law.umaryland.edu/marshall/usccr/documents/cr11042.pdf. Accessed May 6, 2016.

22. *Shelley v Kraemer,* 334 US 1 (1948). Available at: https://supreme.justia.com/cases/federal/us/334/1/case.html. Accessed May 6, 2016.

23. Laskow S. The quiet, massive rezoning of New York. *Politico New York.* February 24, 2014. Available at: http://www.capitalnewyork.com/article/city-hall/2014/02/8540743/quiet-massive-rezoning-new-york?page=all. Accessed March 13, 2016.

24. Brasuell J. Evaluating Bloomberg's massive rezoning efforts. Planetizen: The Urban Planning, Design, and Development Network. February 25, 2014. Available at: http://www.planetizen.com/node/67526. Accessed March 13, 2016.

25. New Yorkers for a Human-Scale City. 2015. Available at: http://www.humanscale.nyc. Accessed March 13, 2016.

26. Richardson JJ. Downzoning, fairness and farmland protection. *J L Use Environ Law.* 2003;19(1):59–90.

27. US Environmental Protection Agency. Smart Growth. 2015. Available at: https://www.epa.gov/smartgrowth. Accessed March 13, 2016.

28. Richardson Jr JJ. Downzoning, fairness and farmland protection. *J Land Use Environ Law.* 2003;19(1):59–90.

29. Jacobs J. *The Death and Life of Great American Cities.* New York, NY: Random House Inc; 1961.

30. *Form-Based Codes: A Step-by-Step Guide for Communities.* Chicago, IL: Chicago Metropolitan Agency for Planning; 2001.

31. US National Park Service. National Register of Historic Places Fundamentals. Available at: https://www.nps.gov/nr/national_register_fundamentals.htm#results. Accessed March 26, 2016.

32. *Establishing Local Historic Districts.* Boston, MA: Massachusetts Historical Commission; 2003.

33. City of Austin Texas. Watershed protection. Available at: http://austintexas.gov/department/watershed-protection. Accessed February 10, 2016.

34. Kotkin J, Piiparinen R. The rustbelt roars back from the dead. *The Daily Beast.* December 7, 2014. Available at: http://www.thedailybeast.com/articles/2014/12/07/the-rustbelt-roars-back-from-the-dead.html. Accessed May 6, 2016.

35. Greenberg MR, Popper FJ, West BM. The TOADS: a new American urban epidemic. *Urban Aff Rev.* 1990;25(3):435–454.

36. Ewing R, Pendall R, Chen D. *Measuring Sprawl and Its Impacts.* Washington, DC: Smart Growth America; 2002.

37. Congress for the New Urbanism. 2015. Available at: https://www.cnu.org. Accessed January 15, 2016.

38. Campbell-Dollaghan K. Celebration, Florida: the utopian town that America just couldn't trust. *Utopia Week.* April 20, 2014. Available at: http://gizmodo.com/celebration-florida-the-utopian-town-that-america-jus-1564479405. Accessed March 26, 2016.

39. Wheeler SM. Sustainability in community development. In: DeFilippis J, Saegert S, eds. *The Community Development Reader*. 2nd ed. New York, NY, and London, England; 2012:175–183.

40. American Planning Association. *Growing Smart Legislative Guidebook*. Available at: https://www.planning.org/growingsmart. Accessed March 22, 2016.

41. Burchell RW, Listokin D, Galley CC. Smart Growth: more than a ghost of urban policy past, less than a bold new horizon. *Hous Policy Debate*. 2000;11(4):821–879.

42. National Association of Realtors. Smart Growth Program Toolkit. 2015. Available at: http://www.realtor.org/programs/smart-growth-program/smart-growth-program-toolkit. Accessed March 27, 2016.

43. Association of State and Territorial Health Officials. Smart Growth Tool Kit. 2016. Available at: http://www.astho.org/Programs/Environmental-Health/Built-and-Synthetic-Environment/Smart-Growth-Tool-Kit. Accessed March 27, 2016.

44. US Environmental Protection Agency. About Smart Growth. 2015. Available at: https://www.epa.gov/smartgrowth/about-smart-growth. Accessed March 13, 2016.

45. US Department of Agriculture. Food Access Research Atlas. 2015. Available at: http://www.ers.usda.gov/data-products/food-access-research-atlas/documentation.aspx. Accessed April 9, 2016.

46. Pothukuchi K, Kaufman JL. The food system: a stranger to the planning field. *J Am Plan Assoc*. 2000;66(2):113–124.

47. Pothukuchi K, Kaufman J. Placing the food system on the urban agenda: the role of municipal institutions in food systems planning. *Agric Human Values*. 1999;16(2):213–224.

48. Schneider D, Rodgers Y van der M, Cheang JM. Local government coordination of community food systems in distressed urban areas. *J Poverty*. 2008;11(4):45–69.

49. Cohen B. Community food security assessment toolkit. US Department of Agriculture. 2002. Available at: https://www.ers.usda.gov/publications/pub-details/?pubid=43179. Accessed May 15, 2017.

50. Fielding JE, Simon PA. Food deserts or food swamps?: Comment on "Fast food restaurants and food stores." *Arch Intern Med*. 2011;171(13):1171–1172.

51. Park H. The most dangerous cities for walking. *New York Times*. August 12, 2011. Available at: http://www.nytimes.com/interactive/2011/08/12/us/most-dangerous-cities-for-walking.html?_r=0. Accessed May 3, 2016.

52. Smart Growth Tulsa. Gallery. Available at: http://smartgrowthtulsa.com/gallery. Accessed March 22, 2017.

53. Brasuell J. Chicago's transit oriented developments becoming more affluent. Planetizen: The Urban Planning, Design, and Development Network. May 2, 2016. Available at: http://www.planetizen.com/node/86061/chicagos-transit-oriented-developments-becoming-more-affluent. Accessed May 3, 2016.

54. Cities with shared bikes. Bike Share. Available at: http://bikeshare.com/map. Accessed May 3, 2016.

55. Fisher M. America's once magical—now mundane—love affair with cars. *Washington Post.* September 2, 2015. Available at: http://www.washingtonpost.com/sf/style/2015/09/02/americas-fading-car-culture. Accessed May 2, 2016.

56. Kriss J. What is green building? 2014. Available at: http://www.usgbc.org/articles/what-green-building. Accessed March 26, 2016.

57. Fannie Mae rewards LEED-certified multifamily properties with a lower interest rate. US Green Building Council. 2015. Available at: http://www.usgbc.org/articles/fannie-mae-rewards-leed-certified-multifamily-properties-lower-interest-rate. Accessed May 2, 2016.

58. Finucane ML, Clancy N, Willis HH, Knopman D. *The Hurricane Sandy Rebuilding Task Force's Infrastructure Resilience Guidelines: An Initial Assessment of Implementation by Federal Agencies.* Santa Monica, CA: Rand Corporation; 2014.

59. National Research Council. *Developing a Framework for Measuring Community Resilience.* Washington, DC: National Academies Press; 2015.

60. US Department of Commerce, National Institute of Standards and Technology. Community resilience planning guide. 2015. Available at: http://www.nist.gov/el/resilience/guide.cfm. Accessed May 10, 2016.

61. US Economic Development Administration. Comprehensive Economic Development Strategy (CEDS) content guidelines. 2016. Available at: https://www.eda.gov/ceds/content/economic-resilience.htm. Accessed May 10, 2016.

62. American Planning Association. Ethical principles in planning. 1992. Available at: https://www.planning.org/ethics/ethicalprinciples.htm. Accessed January 24, 2016.

3

BUILDING BLOCKS OF PUBLIC HEALTH

Defining the Profession

At the outset of this chapter, it is important to distinguish between the traditional definitions of medicine and public health. The Merriam-Webster Dictionary is useful in this regard, defining medicine as "the science and art of dealing with the maintenance and the prevention, alleviation, or cure of disease." By contrast, public health is defined as "the art and science dealing with the protection and improvement of community health by organized community effort and including preventive medicine and sanitary and social science."[1]

Consider that when individuals become ill, they seek out a physician or other clinical care professional to diagnose and treat their condition, not a public health professional. When a group of community members becomes sick with the same disease, or when a common exposure threatens the health of a community, the public health professional is called to the fore. Otherwise stated, medicine focuses on the medical care and prevention needs of the individual whereas public health focuses on the health of a population, whether that population is at the local, state, federal, or global level.

Public health practitioners envision communities where everyone lives a life free of preventable disease, disability, injury, and premature death. They strive to promote healthy behaviors, as well as physical and social environments that promote good health for everyone. These are lofty goals, but they are not new ones. For example, the first issue of the *American Journal of Public Health* includes the presidential address from the 1910 American Public Health Association's (APHA's) 38th annual meeting in Minneapolis, Minnesota. In that address, Charles O. Probst spoke about the global reach of public health, particularly

> the wonderful work of [Walter] Reed and his associates ... who, in discovering the true cause of this dreaded pest [mosquitos] have freed Cuba from a worse fate than Spanish domination [yellow fever].[2]

Probst lauded APHA's Laboratory Section that developed standardized methods for examining air, water, and milk contamination—methods he stated were rapidly being accepted around the globe. He also cited APHA's Section on Vital Statistics for its work with other nations to develop the International Classification of Disease system. At the national level, Probst noted how health problems were linked to the great sociological problems of the day. He advocated "social hygiene" so people could balance work, play, and rest to prevent physical and mental breakdowns. He called for federal laws addressing child labor, as well as laws requiring the teaching of basic hygiene in all public schools.

At the local level, Probst recommended closing dance halls and saloons to remove the temptations that could lead to moral failures and opening playgrounds and more school-houses to better serve the needs of children. Finally, he noted the American Civic Association's aim, "to make living conditions clean and healthful" and the National Municipal League's focus on improving municipal health and sanitation.[3] In summary, the vision for public health presented by the APHA president in 1910 was truly broad, with linkages to biology, social science, statistics, and urban planning at various population levels. Of note is how his recommendations for improving public health were steeped in progressive advocacy.

In the same year as Probst's address, the Flexner Report on Medical Education in the United States and Canada was released under the aegis of the Carnegie Foundation.[4] In that report, Flexner called for setting strict standards for medical education, pointing to the Johns Hopkins University as the model that medical schools should emulate. Shortly after the release of the Flexner Report, the Rockefeller Foundation determined that it would examine education in public health, hosting a conference where the tensions between public health practitioners and academic researchers came to light. In 1915, William Henry Welch and Wickliffe Rose submitted a report to the Rockefeller Foundation on the need for professional public health education, training that would be distinctly separate from that of medical education.[4] Welch, however, clearly favored public health training that would focus on scientific research (based on the German model) whereas Rose preferred training public health professionals who would go into practice (based on the British model).

The Welch–Rose Report led the Rockefeller Foundation to grant Johns Hopkins University the funding necessary to establish the first independent graduate school of public health in the nation. The school's name, School of Hygiene and Public Health, was specifically chosen to reflect both practice and research. Today, many accredited schools and programs in public health continue to recognize this difference in training focus, offering degrees for students intending to practice (MPH, DrPH, or DPH), as well as for students planning their careers around academic research (MS, PhD, or ScD).[5]

Over the past few decades a trend has emerged, renewing the linkages between public health and medicine that existed before separate training pathways for the professions were codified by the Flexner and Welch–Rose Reports. The trend became evident in the 1990s as medical schools began offering joint-degree programs that would allow graduate students to pursue clinical medicine and public health at the same time. Indeed, half of all accredited U.S. medical schools offered joint MD/MPH or DO/MPH programs by 2016.[6] At least one study showed that students receiving joint training in public health and community medicine were more likely to locate in underserved areas,[7] a factor that may aid the nation in achieving a significant public health goal—that of reducing health disparities.[8]

Some of the standard practices of public health a century ago are still applicable today: addressing pest control, controlling the spread of infectious diseases, improving environmental and occupational health, and reducing behavioral health risks for whole populations (smoking cessation, wearing seat belts, etc.). These practices have broadened as new technologies and a better understanding of the health impacts from various types of exposures, as well as some types of public policies, came to light. Some of these achievements must be shared with other disciplines, but they would not have been possible without some basic tools of public health, particularly surveillance and epidemiology, environmental health and safety monitoring, and dogged advocacy for public health programs—tools that would have been easily recognized by the APHA president in 1910.

Organization of Public Health in the United States

When we think about public health, we usually think of the Centers for Disease Control and Prevention (CDC). However, many other federal agencies (e.g., the Department of Agriculture, the Environmental Protection Agency [EPA], the Department of Transportation's National Highway Traffic Safety Administration, and the Department of Labor's Occupational Safety and Health Administration) engage in regulatory activities, research, education, and other types of activities that affect the public's health. Despite all of this involvement, there is no mandate in the U.S. Constitution for the federal government to protect the public's health. That authority lies with the states.

The 50 states and the District of Columbia define their authority over public health through statute, determining which services will be provided, as well as how these services will be organized, financed, and delivered. This means that some functions of public health may be centralized at the state level whereas others may be allocated to other state agencies, county or regional health agencies, or local health departments. In other words, there is no standard model of how public health is organized.

There are more than 2,800 public health departments of various sizes in the United States. Of these, 60 percent serve counties; 18 percent serve a city, town, or township; 11 percent serve a city or county jurisdiction; and 9 percent serve a multicounty region. Nearly half the population of the United States is served by 140 local health departments that serve large jurisdictions (500,000 or more people).[9] Although jurisdictions differ, public health agencies tend to perform the services and activities listed in Table 3.1.

Table 3.1. Services and Activities Typically Performed by State and Local Public Health Agencies

Services and Activities

Disease surveillance, epidemiology, and data collection
- Vital statistics (birth and death records)
- Communicable or infectious disease reports
- Surveys of behavioral risk factors
- Cancer registries
- Childhood immunization registries
- Hospital discharge databases
- Trauma registries
- Epidemiologic activities related to chronic diseases, cancer, environmental threats, and perinatal health

Laboratory services
- Screening newborns for rare genetic abnormalities
- Testing for possible bioterrorism or emerging infectious diseases
- Testing for food-borne illnesses
- Typing influenza virus strains
- Screening children for lead exposure
- Screening people for exposure to environmental toxins
- Testing environmental samples for toxic contaminants

Preparedness and response to public health emergencies
- Specialized disease surveillance
- Laboratory testing
- Outbreak investigations
- Mass prophylaxis
- Quarantine and isolation
- Coordination of emergency medical response

Population-based primary prevention activities
- HIV/AIDS
- Tobacco
- Injuries
- Unintended pregnancy
- Obesity
- Substance abuse
- Violence

Health care services
- Mental health facilities
- Services for children with special needs
- Treatment services for select communicable diseases (e.g., HIV/AIDS and tuberculosis)
- Treatment services for select addictive diseases (e.g., methadone clinics)
- Correctional health
- Monitoring the private-sector delivery system
- Administering certificate of need programs
- Identifying underserved populations
- Regulation of health care providers

(Continued)

Table 3.1. (Continued)

Services and Activities

Regulatory activities (inspecting and licensing)
- Food processing facilities
- Waste removal services
- Correctional facilities
- Laboratory services

Environmental health (detecting and remediating)
- Contaminated food and water
- Radon gas
- Mosquitoes and other disease vectors
- Chemical spills

Surveillance and Epidemiology

Public health surveillance requires gathering information about a population, monitoring that information over time, and evaluating it to identify patterns or trends in the data with epidemiologic methods. The original goal of public health surveillance was to identify infected individuals, quarantine them, and, in so doing, minimize disease transmission.

Quarantine and Quarantine Stations

The earliest use of quarantine in the American colonies was in 1647, when Massachusetts Bay received word that there was a major epidemic of disease in the West Indies. The colony responded by instituting a maritime quarantine of all ships arriving from West Indian ports.[10] Although port cities made efforts to enforce quarantine, a national effort did not begin in the United States until 1878 when thousands of refugees fleeing yellow fever in the Caribbean (mostly Cuba) tried to enter the nation through New Orleans, Louisiana. Widespread fear, along with lobbying from APHA, spurred Congress to pass the National Quarantine Act, which authorized the U.S. Public Health Service (PHS) to collect data on cholera, smallpox, and yellow fever so that states and localities could impose quarantine measures.[11] The Quarantine Act of 1893 further authorized the PHS to collect information on select diseases each week from state and local public health authorities across the nation.[11] By 1901, all states and municipalities reported cases of cholera, smallpox, and tuberculosis to authorities. Some states and cities had additional reporting requirements so that cases of diseases such as typhoid could be identified and isolated.[12,13]

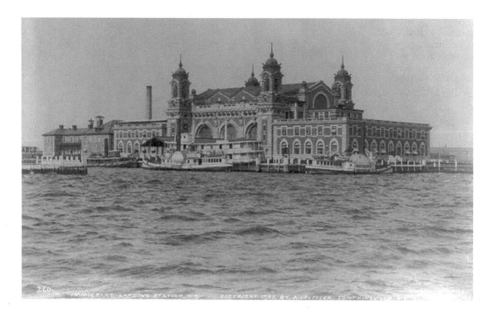

Source: Reprinted from Library of Congress.[14]
Figure 3.1. Ellis Island in 1905

Overwhelmed by mass immigration in the latter half of the 19th and early 20th centuries, local authorities slowly but surely turned over responsibility for screening immigrants at quarantine stations to the federal government. This shift made places such as Ellis Island the main point of entry for most immigrants (Figure 3.1). Records show that about 12 million immigrants entered through Ellis Island between 1892 and 1954. Once on the island, they passed through a line of physicians who would quickly evaluate each one to see if they coughed, wheezed, or limped. Infectious diseases that could lead to an applicant being iso-lated and deported were cholera, trachoma, and tuberculosis. Other diseases that could lead to deportation included insanity, epilepsy, and mental impairments. The system was fast, if imperfect, resulting in the majority of immigrants being allowed to enter with only 1 percent turned away.[15] Today, the massive structure at Ellis Island has been restored and reopened as the Ellis Island National Museum of Immigration, hosting about 2 million visitors annually.[16]

Large quarantine stations have gone the way of the dinosaur, but small ones remain. Before September 11, 2001, the United States had eight remaining quarantine stations. After the attacks, fears of bioterrorism and the global outbreak of severe acute respiratory syndrome (SARS) led the CDC to open 20 quarantine stations. These are located at the following points of entry and land border crossings:

- Anchorage, Alaska
- Atlanta, Georgia
- Boston, Massachusetts

- Chicago, Illinois
- Dallas, Texas
- Detroit, Michigan
- El Paso, Texas
- Honolulu, Hawaii
- Houston, Texas
- Los Angeles, California
- Miami, Florida
- Minneapolis, Minnesota
- Newark, New Jersey
- New York, New York
- Philadelphia, Pennsylvania
- San Diego, California
- San Francisco, California
- San Juan, Puerto Rico
- Seattle, Washington
- Washington, District of Columbia

Isolation is defined as separating individuals who are ill from those who are not. Quarantine differs from isolation as it both separates and restricts the movements of individuals who have been exposed to a communicable (contagious; able to be passed from person-to-person) disease to see if they develop it. The federal government derives its authority to restrict the movement of individuals who may not be sick, including those who may be U.S. citizens, from Section 361 of the Public Health Service Act (42 U.S. Code § 264). That act gives the U.S. Secretary of Health and Human Services the authority to take measures to prevent the entry and spread of communicable diseases from foreign countries into the United States and between states.[17]

Today's 20 quarantine stations are staffed 24 hours a day, seven days a week by quarantine officers who perform various types of duties. They respond to reports of illnesses, screen cargo and inspect animals and animal products for disease, and monitor the health and collect medical information on new immigrants, refugees, parolees, and individuals seeking asylum. Quarantine officers have the authority to detain or refuse entry to anyone suspected of having or developing a contagious disease on the quarantine list. On July 31, 2014, President Barack Obama issued an executive order[18] updating that list as follows:

- Cholera
- Diphtheria
- Infectious tuberculosis
- Plague
- Smallpox

- Yellow fever
- Viral hemorrhagic fevers
- Severe acute respiratory syndrome
- New types of flu (influenza) that could cause a pandemic

The second author of this book had a first-hand experience with the quarantine station at Newark, New Jersey, many decades ago, before smallpox was declared globally eradicated in 1979. She was returning home from traveling abroad but forgot to pack her immunization papers along with her passport. A quarantine officer removed her from the immigration line and took her to the quarantine station where she was asked to remove her arm from her sleeve and show him her smallpox vaccination scar. Unfortunately, she did not have one. This created quite a stir and several other individuals were called in to examine both of her arms carefully for a scar. They found none. The staff of the quarantine station spent about five minutes discussing the issue before announcing to her that she would have to be immunized against smallpox on the spot. If not, she would not be able to return home. Up went the sleeve, in went the vaccine, and the author was on her way home. As with the first smallpox immunization, she never developed a scar.

Not everyone who may have been exposed to a disease on the quarantine list may have had such a simple outcome. Consider the case of Kaci Hickox, a 34-year-old nurse who served with Doctors Without Borders in a valiant effort to contain the Ebola outbreak in Sierra Leone. On her return trip in 2014, Hickox landed at Newark Airport on her way home to Maine. There she was quarantined under a policy that had just been put into place under governors Chris Christie of New Jersey and Andrew Cuomo of New York. The new policy required all arriving air travelers who had contact with Ebola patients in West Africa to be quarantined for 21 days, the maximum incubation period for the disease. Medical experts and the White House strongly criticized the action, as it was considerably stricter than the guidelines for quarantine developed by the CDC. Hickox was held in a quarantine tent in an unheated parking garage at University Hospital in Newark, where she had access to a portable toilet but no running water. She had to request blankets and had to speak to people through a plastic window. After two days and massive media criticism, the nurse was allowed to continue her trip home. Once in Maine, a judge ruled she need not be restricted to her home as long as she kept health officials apprised of any symptoms she might develop.[19] Hickox's experience with quarantine raises some important questions:

- What is appropriate practice when science is unable to rule out theoretical disease transmission risks?
- How much power should states have to quarantine individuals to protect population health?
- How do we respect individual liberty while still using the best epidemiologic data to set public health policy?

Monitor and Control Infectious Diseases

Many diseases that threaten the public's health are communicable, but they are not on today's quarantine list because immunizations or treatments are now available. It is also important to note that although all communicable diseases are infectious, not all infectious diseases are communicable. Specifically, infectious diseases are caused by microorganisms (bacteria, viruses, parasites, or fungi) and can be spread through contaminated food (such as botulism), water (such as cholera), or the general environment (such as tetanus). They can also be spread through contact with animals (such as rabies) or insect bites (such as malaria), or from person to person (such as influenza). Infectious diseases that transmit from animals to humans are called zoonotic diseases. Those that transmit from human to human through direct or indirect contact are termed communicable diseases.

Not all communicable diseases are vaccine-preventable at the time of the outbreak and quarantine may be the only solution, particularly when asymptomatic carriers threaten the population. Consider the story of Irish immigrant Mary Mallon (nicknamed "Typhoid Mary") who worked as a cook for affluent families in New York City from 1900 to 1907. Mallon's time with each family was short as residents of the households she served became seriously ill with typhoid fever within two to three weeks of her employ. The cook freely admitted to poor personal hygiene, but she refused to believe she was the cause of illness because she herself was not ill. As there was neither vaccine nor treatment available for typhoid at the time, city health inspector Dr. Josephine Baker took Mallon into custody and quarantined her on North Brother Island for two years. Mallon was then released on the sole condition that she would no longer work as a cook. After working as a laundress for two years, the asymptomatic typhoid carrier changed her name and returned to her former occupation. Mallon was re-arrested in 1915 after starting an epidemic of typhoid at Sloan Hospital for Women in Manhattan where she worked as a cook. The remainder of her life was spent in quarantine at Riverside Hospital, where she died at age 69. The number of cases of typhoid she left in her wake is unknown, but multiple sources estimate that Mallon caused at least 50 deaths.

The story of Mary Mallon shows that not all communicable diseases can be controlled through case identification and isolation. Some can only be controlled through vaccine programs and public policies that enforce immunizations for public school attendance. Polio, for example, can only be controlled through immunization. Immunization programs and mandatory immunization policies are not without critics, however, a situation that can be traced back to the roots of the nation, as the following smallpox illustration demonstrates.

The American story of immunization begins in colonial Boston, Massachusetts, a city that suffered multiple smallpox epidemics between 1640 and 1721 in which hundreds of residents lost their lives. While the practice of smallpox inoculation (variolation) was known if not understood, religious faith opposed the practice. The community was split, with two prominent Bostonians, Reverend Cotton Mather and physician Zabdiel Boylston, taking a pro-inoculation stance. Local physician William Douglass led those in opposition. Despite severe criticism and a war of words in local newspapers,[20] Boylston undertook an experiment by smearing pus from active smallpox lesions into small wounds made into three healthy individuals—an adult slave (Jack), a two-year-old slave (Jackey), and Boylston's own six-year-old son. All three developed mild cases of small-pox, but all survived and demonstrated lifelong immunity from the disease. Boylston's experiment led some Bostonians to agree to become inoculated, but far more refused. The physician later compared data on future smallpox outbreaks in Boston, reporting that mortality from smallpox was about 2 percent among those inoculated compared with about 15 percent among those who were not.[21]

The commander of the Continental Army, George Washington, ordered the first large-scale mandatory immunization program in the colonies. Smallpox not only rav-aged the Native American population, but it also threatened to destroy the fighting power of Washington's troops during the Revolutionary War. John Adams wrote of this problem in a letter to his wife, Abigail, in 1776:

> The smallpox is ten times more terrible than the British, Canadians, and Indians together. This was the cause of our precipitate retreat from Quebec.[22]

Outbreaks of smallpox happened routinely in the coastal cities of Boston, Philadelphia, and Charleston, South Carolina, but most of Washington's soldiers were from the interior and had no experience with the disease. As the general could not afford to have his fight-ing men down with this contagion, nor could he have survivors recuperating for up to one month, he issued two orders. First, no soldier in the Continental Army was allowed to be inoculated (live virus was used at that time), as even a mild case of smallpox would rapidly spread through the troops. Second, he ordered mandatory inoculation of any new recruit who had no previous immunity to the disease. This way, new recruits under-going outfitting and training would contract a milder form of smallpox and become immune before joining the fighting ranks. Thus, Washington's Continental Army was the first in the world to undergo an organized military inoculation program against a com-municable disease.[23]

Even when vaccines become available, the level of immunization in the popula-tion (herd immunity) may not be high enough to prevent outbreaks. For instance, 667 cases of measles were reported in the United States in 2014, the majority of whom were not vaccinated for the disease.[24] Public health authorities continue to struggle with individual and community resistance to vaccine programs, resistance not terribly dissimilar from the resistance faced by Mather and Boylston in colonial Boston.

Surveillance

The story of surveillance to estimate total population health begins in 1921, when the PHS launched the Hagerstown [Maryland] Morbidity Survey. The survey was spearheaded by Edgar Sydenstricker, chief of the agency's Office of Statistical Investigations, who argued: "Statistics of illness can afford an indication of [population] vitality ... more illuminating than mortality."[25] These words were particularly meaningful as the United States entered the second half of the 20th century and noninfectious diseases took more American lives than did infectious ones. Diabetes, as well as liver, kidney, and cardiovascular diseases, placed a new and significant burden on the overall health of the population. To understand the scope of the issue, the National Health Interview Survey (NHIS) was launched in 1957. The systematic and continued collection of NHIS survey data today allows epidemiologists to examine the way health outcomes differ according to time (days, months, or years), place (geographic area), and characteristics of persons (Table 3.2).

Epidemiologists use the information from population-based health surveys along with other data to determine associations between risk factors and various health outcomes. Examples of these associations include cigarette smoking as a risk factor for

Table 3.2. Characteristics of Persons Evaluated by Epidemiologists

Demographic characteristics
- Age
- Gender
- Race
- Ethnic group

Biological characteristics
- Levels of antibodies, chemicals, and enzymes
- Blood constituents such as cells and platelets
- Measures of organ and systems function such as blood glucose or hormone levels

Social and economic characteristics
- Socioeconomic status
- Educational background
- Occupation
- Place of birth

Behavioral factors
- Tobacco, alcohol, and drug use
- Diet
- Physical exercise

Genetic factors
- Blood groups
- Gene mutations

Source: Based on Schneider and Lilienfeld.[26]

lung cancer and obesity as a risk factor for diabetes. Epidemiologists also use these types of data to monitor disease prevention and control efforts, such as whether fewer people smoke after the launch of antismoking campaigns or whether the rate of obesity declines after changes in nutritional recommendations. Information from population-based surveys can also be used to determine the health impacts of public policies such instituting a minimum age for the purchase of cigarettes or requiring dietary labels on food packaging. Otherwise stated, population-based surveys provide the information needed for understanding the overall burden of disease on the population and how that burden changes over time.

Syndromic Surveillance

Before September 11, 2001, monitoring population health and reporting new cases of notifiable diseases as soon as they were diagnosed was standard practice for public health surveillance. After that date, it became clear that we needed more rapid reporting of some types of health outcomes. The answer to the need was syndromic surveillance, a system tied to real-time reporting. Syndromic surveillance identifies potential cases, not simply already diagnosed ones. A potential case might be an individual exposed or suspected to have been exposed to a bioterrorist agent (anthrax, radiation), or one who has only minor or early symptoms of a disease such as influenza, which is not yet diagnosed. By shortening the time to case identification in emergency situations, impacted individuals may be isolated and, if possible, treated early in order to save their lives and protect the general public from disease spread.[27]

How can cases be found before they have been diagnosed? Many, particularly larger, hospital emergency departments now have real time reporting links to centralized servers linked to public health agencies. When a patient is seen in these facilities, their symptoms are entered into an electronic health record and a message is automatically sent to local, state, and national public health agencies for monitoring. If cases with similar symptoms (or diagnoses) appear, even if they present to different hospitals, a red flag is tripped and an investigation may ensue.[28] Similarly, prescription drug sales in some cities and states are monitored electronically, as are some over-the-counter medicines that are bar-coded and scanned at the point of sale in larger pharmacies and supermarkets. An increase in sales of antibiotics, or sales of over-the-counter medications for fever or diarrhea, can quickly send up a red flag for public health authorities to investigate.

The World Health Organization (WHO) has international health syndromic surveillance reporting requirements for its 194 member states. WHO requires that it be notified of any public health event of potential international importance, even if the causative agent is not yet known.[29] By reducing the time between exposure and diagnosis, real-time reporting allows for a rapid public health response to a bioterrorist event (such as radiation exposure or inhalational anthrax), as well as new and re-emerging diseases that may not be readily identified but pose serious regional or global threats (such as Ebola or Zika virus).

Sentinel Surveillance

One of the ways that public health tries to keep ahead of disease outbreaks, particularly at the local level, is through sentinel surveillance. Sentinel surveillance relies on the first (sentinel) health event or environmental indicator that allows public health professionals to know that prevention efforts or medical care needs to be improved. Consider these sentinel events:

1. Assume a first (sentinel) case of measles is reported by the nurse at a local school. That first case indicates the immediate need for attention to immunizations and public health goes into overdrive. The state public health agency is notified and the case is reported to the National Notifiable Diseases Surveillance System. A letter or email is sent home to parents explaining the dangers of the disease and asking them to be sure their child is immunized. The school nurse reviews immunization records to identify children at risk. Public health and local media report information on symptoms to look for so that those with or likely to develop the disease are isolated at home. Other vulnerable individuals may choose to restrict their movements in public places to minimize their risk of exposure. Usually, the outbreak is quickly contained.

2. Assume a bicyclist is out for a morning ride and sees a dead crow alongside the road, something the bicyclist has not seen on any other morning rides (a sentinel event). The bicyclist calls the local health department who dispatches a worker to use gloves to retrieve the dead crow for analysis. The concern about the dead crow is that it may signal the arrival of West Nile virus in the community. While waiting for the state laboratory results, public health officials issue local media releases, encouraging residents to use insect repellent and wear protective clothing when outdoors. They may also call the appropriate state agency to discuss a spraying program to reduce the local mosquito population.

3. Consider that a worker at a local factory has developed a rare form of cancer, one that has been linked to occupational exposures. This (sentinel) care of a rare disease will be reported to the state cancer registry and the Occupational Safety and Health Administration (OSHA) may be called. An investigation into the workplace may ensue whereby environmental health specialists will determine exposure levels to potential carcinogens throughout the workplace and epidemiologists may examine work records to estimate duration of exposure risk(s). OSHA may

require management to provide the workers with protective gear, make changes to processes or equipment to protect workers from toxic or carcinogenic exposures, or (if warranted) pose fines sufficient to close the facility if the risk to workers is an imminent threat.

Sentinel surveillance may include biomonitoring, particularly of sentinel animals or insect vectors. Chickens have been used as sentinel animals to determine the presence of West Nile virus in places as varied as Senegal,[30] Greece,[31] and California.[32] The chickens are maintained in locations where they are likely to be exposed to mosquitos and their blood is drawn on a regular basis to determine if they have developed antibodies to the disease. Similarly, dogs have been used as sentinel animals to estimate the burden of zoonotic parasites among indigenous populations.[33] Both companion and working dogs are tested for parasites that also infect humans and, when found in the sentinel animals, both the dogs and the humans they live with are treated.

Americans tend to forget that the nation suffered epidemics of yellow fever not all that long ago. The risk was significantly reduced when we drained swamps, installed sewers to channel runoff, and began sleeping in residences with screens on the windows. A massive spraying program also helped, but the native mosquito species capable of carrying the disease never disappeared and some recently introduced species have added to our mosquito burden. For example, mosquitos inhabit international shipping containers and are transported worldwide for international trade. Of great concern is the Asian tiger mosquito, which is highly adapted to urban and suburban areas. These mosquitos, along with other species, have been implicated as the vectors of new and re-emerging diseases in the United States, particularly dengue, chikungunya, and Zika.[34]

Strategically placed mosquito traps allow entomologists and mosquito control workers to capture, sort, and identify various species of mosquitos that land in the traps. When the species that transmit new and re-emerging diseases are identified in an area (a sentinel event), public health messages can be issued that encourage individuals to take precautions against being bitten and trigger spraying campaigns to protect the general public.

Monitoring sentinel insect vectors is vitally important as outbreaks of the diseases they carry have global implications. For example, in February 2016, WHO declared that the cluster of cases of Zika virus in Brazil presented a public health emergency of international concern.[35] Discussions of what this meant for the Summer Olympic Games in Rio de Janeiro began to circulate immediately. In June 2016, Julie Beck wrote a story for *The Atlantic* asking, "Should the Olympics be postponed because of Zika?"[36] Beck reported that more than 200 physicians, bioethicists, and public health specialists had posted on open letter online calling for the games to be postponed or moved "in the name of public health."

By July, travel-related cases of Zika were reported in Florida.[37] Mosquito monitoring was increased and the sentinel species that carry the disease was identified in a Miami neighborhood. The CDC responded by issuing a warning about travel to that neighborhood and the impacts on the Florida tourist economy were immediate. Travelers canceled their vacation plans and Bloomberg News reported that the state's tourist industry could lose $90 billion.[38] CBS News reported that while Florida was spending millions on mosquito control, funding at the federal level had stalled for political reasons. The article went on to explain that the birth of even one child with microcephaly because of a pregnant woman being exposed to Zika would cost about $10 million for lifetime medical and supportive care. Indeed, failure to invest in public health prevention measures when they are called for by effective surveillance is penny-wise and pound-foolish.

Environmental Health

The purpose of environmental health is to identify and remediate conditions that endanger the health of populations. Did you get sick after eating at a local restaurant? Does your tap water smell bad or does it have a brown or black color? Did you see a rat near the empty house at the end of the street? Perhaps noise from the airport keeps you up all night. If so, you will likely call your local health department where an environmental health and safety specialist will be dispatched to look into the issue.

Environmental health professionals often aid residents in identifying problems and suggesting solutions for their homes, such as how to deal with bedbug infestations, high levels of radon, and the cleanup of mold and fungus after storms and floods. They may be dispatched to investigate outbreaks of disease at the local level, such as a foodborne illness after a local event, or an outbreak of head lice from contaminated naptime cots at a nursery school. We have already described how public health surveillance includes monitoring disease vectors, particularly mosquitos, ticks, rats, and rabid animals. Once identified, environmental health professionals are often called upon to perform pest-control functions.

Environmental health measures to control insect-borne diseases began more than a century ago when Walter Reed's U.S. Army Yellow Fever Commission reported that the disease was carried by mosquitos and instituted measures such as draining swamps, cutting back brush, and more.[39] With the development of chemical pesticides in the early 20th century (particularly DDT), control of mosquitoes and other insect vectors became common worldwide. Despite the overuse of some of these agents and their legacy, chemical and bio-pesticides remain important tools to protect the public from diseases such as Lyme disease, eastern equine encephalitis, Rocky Mountain spotted fever, West Nile virus, and more. Despite aggressive efforts at controlling these vectors, almost half a million Americans are stricken by insect-borne illnesses each year.[40]

Environmental health and safety professionals monitor indoor and outdoor air quality, public and private potable water supplies, and both solid waste and onsite sewage disposal systems. They perform inspections of food service locations and public recreational facilities, closing down those that put the public at risk until problems can be remediated. Perhaps lesser known is that environmental health and safety specialists inspect pet shops and kennels, tanning and tattooing parlors, daycare centers and nursing homes, and children's camps and playgrounds. Some even investigate and seek remediation of local nuisances, such as the presence of poison ivy, garbage, or dangerous housing conditions.

The authors have worked with environmental health professionals for years, serving on investigatory teams charged with looking into exposures that might contribute to adverse health effects in communities. As an example, the second author traveled to a poor community in the Deep South where the residents were concerned about serious health outcomes, particularly cancer. The local population believed their poor health was the result of the presence of a large facility a dozen miles away that received and processed toxic waste. After checking in to the only motel in the county (without a TV and with several spiders in the shower), touring the facility of concern, participating in public meetings, and trying desperately to find a green vegetable on a menu anywhere in a local restaurant, the problem became clear. The community's poor health was rooted in poverty, poor nutrition and obesity, smoking, and lack of access to preventive medical and dental care. No exposure route could be identified from the toxic waste facility.

Occupational Health and Safety

Environmental health professionals in both the community and private sectors often also hold positions designed to protect workers from dangerous working conditions and exposures. We have been privileged to participate in some of these efforts. For example, the second author participated in an occupational health and safety investigation for migrant workers in the chili fields in El Paso, Texas. That investigation was instigated by a community health organization and yielded interesting results—particularly that exposure to chemicals was less of a health threat than the workers' everyday working conditions.[41]

We began our investigation by surveying more than 800 El Paso migrant workers in English and Spanish. The data showed that the workers were predominantly Hispanic, with a mean age of 51 years, and typically with 18 years of experience in agriculture (mostly with chilies). The workers averaged 7.2 hours each day in the field. Only 8 percent of the workers reported being exposed to pesticides, and laboratory testing of their clothing showed that pesticide exposures were not significant. It is possible that this low number of exposures to pesticides was a reflection of improved training and caution taken by the workers.

Our on-site investigations of field conditions showed multiple problems with limited access to food, water, and hygiene opportunities. While most of the workers had access to drinking water (97 percent), 20 percent of them did not have access to food during the working day. We were somewhat surprised that 30 percent of them were offered alcohol for purchase on their breaks and at the end of the day. Almost one-third of the workers did not have water available for hand washing after using portable toilets in the fields. Our investigation provided local advocacy groups with the data they needed to pressure state and federal agencies to enforce existing regulations to protect these migrant workers.

Occupational health and safety overlaps with the field of industrial hygiene as both professions monitor job sites to be sure that appropriate health and safety measures are followed. Industrial hygienists are trained in anatomy and physiology, as well as in understanding the damage that various biological, chemical, ergonomic, physical, and radiation exposures can cause to the human body. Industrial hygienists observe workflow and production processes, using checklists and surveys (see Chapter 5) to better understand workers' perceptions of their jobs. Finally, they use monitoring devices (air, noise, radiation, and more) to obtain and analyze data to determine whether any changes need to be made to protect the health of the workers. Although industrial hygienists mostly hold master's degrees or higher, not all environmental health workers are required to hold college degrees.

Sanitation and Hazardous Waste Materials

We do not typically think of sanitation workers as part of the public health workforce, but their efforts to keep our communities clean and disease-free are critical to environmental health.[42] Sanitation workers not only pick up residential and commercial trash, but they also are charged with transporting and disposing of it properly. Garbage, recycled materials, and hazardous items should be collected and disposed of separately. Indeed, many municipalities set special pickup dates or drop-off sites for items such as batteries, chemicals, electronics, paint, pesticides, and others. Industries often have special pick-up services to deal with these items.

When the disposal of hazardous items and/or waste products is difficult or costly, the items may wind up dumped in places where they endanger public health and the environment. Individuals, communities, industry, and the government have been guilty of these dumping practices, leaving behind a legacy of actual or potential toxic disasters. Three events clearly awoke the public to the problem:

1. During World War II, the Hanford Site along the Columbia River in Washington accumulated hazardous waste from the construction of the atomic bomb. The facility

continued to make plutonium for five decades, leaving a huge nuclear cleanup problem. The cleanup at Hanford continues, with estimated costs projected beyond $100 billion, and will continue until 2060 or 2070.[43] The same problem exists, although at a lesser extent, at Department of Energy sites at Savannah River (South Carolina), Oak Ridge (Tennessee), and Idaho Falls (Idaho; see Chapter 8 for a case study of the Fernald Preserve, Ohio, a Comprehensive Environmental Response, Compensation, and Liability Act, or CERCLA, site).

2. In 1978, residents of the Love Canal neighborhood of Niagara Falls, New York, suffered significant health problems that were traced to the Hooker Chemical Company's dumping of chemical and toxic wastes into the abandoned canal. The cleanup took 21 years and cost $400 million.[44] Very little of the area has been redeveloped.

3. In 1978, a 23-acre site near Louisville, Kentucky, was found to have received more than 100,000 drums of toxic waste, 27,000 of which were buried and the others dumped directly into pits or trenches. The owner had died and no one claimed the property. The EPA declared the site an emergency as high levels of heavy metals, polychlorinated biphenyls, and 140 other chemicals were contaminating local waterways and the aquifer. The site took seven years to clean up with an estimated cost of about $4 million.[45]

These events spurred federal legislative action beginning in 1976. Two programs to deal with the cleanup of toxic wastes were implemented: (1) CERCLA (or Superfund), which was designed to deal with the cleanup of existing waste sites, and (2) the Resource Conservation and Recovery Act, designed to address newly generated hazardous wastes.

With the legislation in place, the number of places requiring cleanup of toxic materials required a new and specially trained workforce. OSHA, along with the U.S. Coast Guard, the National Institute for Occupational Safety and Health, and the EPA, developed Hazardous Waste Operations and Emergency Response standards to protect these workers. Hazardous materials (HAZMAT) workers participate in the emergency response to the release of, or threat of release of, hazardous substances. They are required to complete special trainings to be licensed to work with some hazardous materials, particularly asbestos and lead. More extensive training is required to work at nuclear facilities.

We were interested in seeing how many hazardous waste sites were in our area, so we logged on to TOXMAP.[46] This interactive mapping program allows the user to explore various EPA databases by location. We typed in our campus address and found a facility on the Toxic Release Inventory (TRI) list within 1 mile of our offices. A slight zoom out and we found six TRI facilities and one cleaned-up Superfund site within 2.5 miles. The site is fun to use and may be an eye opener for some (see Chapter 11 for a view of the EPA Web site and discussion of some of its tools, as well as Chapter 7).

Public Health Emergency Preparedness

Environmental health reaches into public health emergency preparedness (PHEP), working with first responders and multiple layers of government to plan for, react to, and help populations recover from disasters. Although the nation was prepared to respond to hurricanes and floods before September 11, 2001, the 9/11 attacks, along with the anthrax crisis that followed shortly thereafter, spurred Congress to invest in PHEP. One of the more accepted definitions of PHEP is

> the capability of the public health and health care systems, communities, and individuals, to prevent, protect against, quickly respond to, and recover from health emergencies, particularly those whose scale, timing, or unpredictability threatens to overwhelm routine capabilities.[47]

PHEP is a clear arena in which public health and planning must interact. Key elements of PHEP are shown in Table 3.3.

In 2006, the Pandemic and All-Hazards Preparedness Act established a new position, Assistant Secretary for Preparedness and Response, within the Department of Health and Human Services. The Assistant Secretary was given the authority to develop programs, including advanced development of medical countermeasures, and charged with a quadrennial National Health Security Strategy (NHSS). The strategic objectives of the NHSS are as follows:

1. Build and sustain healthy, resilient communities.
2. Enhance the national capability to produce and effectively use medical countermeasures and nonpharmaceutical interventions.
3. Ensure comprehensive health situational awareness to support decision-making before incidence and during response and recovery operations.
4. Enhance the integration and effectiveness of the public health, health care, and emergency management systems.
5. Strengthen global health security.[48]

Note the overlap in the vocabulary used by the planning and public health professions in the first strategic objective. This shared vocabulary appears again in the second bullet in the following list when in 2011 the CDC defined a set of public health preparedness capabilities:

- Biosurveillance
- Community resilience
- Countermeasures and mitigation
- Incident management
- Information management[49]

Table 3.3. Elements of Public Health Preparedness

Pre-planned and coordinated rapid-response capability
- Health risk assessment (identify and address the needs of high-risk populations, structures, and industries)
- Legal climate (understand liability and the ability to impose restrictions on movement of persons, enforce professional credentialing)
- Roles and responsibilities (define the roles of police, emergency medical services, public health, health care facilities, and others within and across jurisdictions)
- Incident command system (keep responders abreast of their functions with an integrated system)
- Public health engagement (keep the public educated and informed so they can be active participants in public health emergency preparedness)
- Epidemiology functions (monitor, detect, and investigate potential hazards)
- Laboratory functions (maintain and update capacity to address environmental, radiological, toxic, or infectious hazards)
- Countermeasures and mitigation strategies (prepare for mass distribution of medications and vaccines, and establish the capability for isolation and quarantine)
- Mass health care (address "hospital search" and employ field medical stations and other venues as needed)
- Public information and communication (use risk communication strategies for targeted and culturally appropriate messages, build these skills among spokespersons before the emergency)
- Robust supply chain (develop public and private partnerships drawing upon the expertise of the military, business, and other partners with experience in supply chain)

Expert and fully staffed workforce
- Operations-ready workers and volunteers (train and test staff to perform optimally under stressful circumstances)
- Leadership (place emphasis on the training, recruitment, and development of public health leaders)

Accountability and quality improvement
- Testing operational capabilities (use exercises, drills, and real events to assess performance and make improvements)
- Performance management (use clear performance measures to provide data that can be used for quality improvement and close performance gaps)
- Financial tracking (develop, test, and improve financial systems to track resources and ensure adequate and timely reimbursement of third parties during an emergency)

Source: Based on Nelson et al. 2008.[47]

The tasks of PHEP have since expanded. Jurisdictions must now be able to respond to aspects of animal disease, food and agriculture safety, and environmental health, as well as to chemical, biological, radiological, nuclear, and explosive events. They must still address vulnerable populations, and they must still help communities plan for resilience. To do that, PHEP must utilize all of the resources in the community, engaging not only first responders, medical personnel, and public health workers but also planners and the community at large.

Advocacy and Public Policy

Major public health organizations such as APHA, the National Association of County and City Health Officials (NACCHO), and the Society of Public Health Educators (SOPHE) play advocacy roles for changing or instituting new local, state, and national policies and legislation to improve community health. For instance, APHA claims its main advocacy concerns are (1) ensuring access to care, (2) protecting funding for core public health programs and services, and (3) eliminating health disparities.[50] The organization's advocacy Web page asserts that it is also working on the following:

- Emergency preparedness
- Food safety
- Hunger and nutrition
- Climate change and other environmental health issues
- Public health infrastructure
- Disease control
- International health
- Tobacco control

NACCHO has an expansive advocacy Web site containing all of its policy statements and communications to both Congress and the administration.[51] Separate Web pages with links to each are provided for the following topical areas (also see Chapter 11 for more on the NACCHO site):

- Community health (e.g., access to health services, chronic disease prevention, immunization, healthy community design, infectious disease and epidemiology, injury and violence prevention, maternal and child health, tobacco).
- Environmental health (e.g., environmental hazards, justice, and policy; food safety).
- Public health infrastructure (e.g., health and social justice, health information technology, quality improvement, workforce development).
- Public health preparedness (e.g., community resilience, medical countermeasures and nonpharmaceutical interventions, public health and health care systems preparedness, global health security).

Public health educators share a vision of promoting quality of life and healthy behaviors by developing, implementing, and evaluating health education programs. They are committed to addressing issues such as addictive behaviors, violence prevention, physical activity, and social engagement. As the main professional organization for public health educators, SOPHE requires public health advocacy of its members. The organization's advocacy Web page states:

> Advocating for public health policies is part of SOPHE's mission as a health education organization. SOPHE has a responsibility to educate decision-makers on national and state legislative issues related to a healthy society.[52]

In consort with this mission, SOPHE hosts an Annual Advocacy Summit, a three-day event during which the first two days provide advocacy training and the third day requires a visit with legislators or their key staff on Capitol Hill.

Achieve Health Equity

There are federal programs designed to ensure that all citizens have access to adequate health care and nutrition, including the Affordable Care Act; Medicare; the Special Supplemental Nutrition Program for Women, Infants and Children; and more. States, localities, and community-based organizations also fund programs such as food banks, free clinics, Meals on Wheels, senior centers, and visiting nurse services. It is undeniable that these and other programs have helped remove barriers to accessing adequate amounts of nutritious food and basic health care, but the data show that there are still disparities in health outcomes for large portions of the population, particularly minority groups.

The Healthy People 2020 initiative spearheaded by the CDC defines health equity and related terms:

- Health equity: Attainment of the highest level of health for all people. Health equity means efforts to ensure that all people have full and equal access to opportunities that enable them to lead healthy lives.
- Health inequalities: Differences in health that are avoidable, unfair, and unjust. Health inequities are affected by social, economic, and environmental conditions.
- Health disparities: Differences in health outcomes among groups of people.[53]

The Web site provides a tool to help public health practitioners understand the data on health disparities, particularly differences in outcomes based on sex, race/ethnicity, educational attainment, and socioeconomic status. The CDC points out that age, disability, sexual identity, and geographic location also contribute to an individual's ability to achieve good health.

The APHA takes a slightly different (albeit complementary) approach to achieving health equity. The organization's Web site asserts that health equity is a guiding principle and a core value of the organization. Note how many of the items in the APHA statement below overlap with those that concern the planning profession:

> We value all people equally. We optimize the conditions in which people are born, grow, live, work, learn and age. We work with other sectors to address the factors that influence health, including employment, housing, education, health care, public safety and food access. We name racism as a force in determining how these social determinants are distributed.[54]

In 2014, the Robert Wood Johnson (RWJ) Foundation began issuing awards to reduce health disparities and achieve health equity. The RWJ Foundation's Web site is clear that it seeks a shakeup of established systems because many health disparities are caused by non-medical determinants of health. To begin the shakeup, the RWJ Foundation funded non-profit organizations that would champion systems change. Funding opportunities have since been opened to business organizations, media, and faith-based and philanthropic organizations with a track record of seeking systems change that will influence "access to quality health care, education, employment, income, community, environment, housing or public safety."[55]

The future for public health and planning professionals to work together has never been brighter and is essential to protect human health and safety. Chapter 2 pointed out that the professions already share use of the same population-based data sets, public survey results, statistical software packages, and other tools designed for working with communities. We can use these common tools, as well as others presented in the coming chapters, to shake up established systems and achieve health equity (both population and environmental health equity) for all.

References

1. Medicine. *Merriam-Webster Dictionary*. Available at: http://www.merriam-webster.com/dictionary/medicine. Accessed January 18, 2016.

2. Probst CO. President's address. *Am J Public Health*. 1911;1(1):10–20.

3. Welch W, Rose W. *Institute of Hygiene: Presented to the General Education Board*. New York, NY: The Rockefeller Foundation; 1915.

4. Flexner A. *Medical Education in the United States and Canada: A Report to the Carnegie Foundation for the Advancement of Teaching*. New York, NY: The Carnegie Foundation for the Advancement of Teaching; 1910.

5. Lee JM, Furner SE, Yager J, Hoffman D. A review of the status of the doctor of public health degree and identification of future issues. *Public Health Rep*. 2009;124(1):177–183.

6. American Association of Medical Colleges. Directory of MD–MPH Educational Opportunities. 2016. Available at: https://students-residents.aamc.org/applying-medical-school/article/directory-md-mph-educational-opportunities. Accessed March 3, 2017.

7. Xierali IM, Maeshiro R, Johnson S, Arceneaux T, Fair MA. Public health and community medicine instruction and physician practice location. *Am J Prev Med*. 2014;47(5 suppl 3):S297–S300.

8. Healthy People 2020. About Healthy People. Available at: http://www.healthypeople.gov/2020/About-Healthy-People. Accessed January 18, 2016.

9. *2008 National Profile of Local Health Departments*. Washington, DC: National Association of County and City Health Officials; 2008.

10. Parmet WE. Health care and the Constitution: public health and the role of the state in the framing era. *Hastings Constit Law Q*. 1993;20(2):267–335.

11. Michael JM. The National Board of Health: 1879–1883. *Public Health Rep*. 2011;126(1):123–129.

12. Leavitt JW. *Typhoid Mary: Captive to the Public's Health*. 10th ed. Boston, MA: Beacon Press; 1997.

13. Soper GA. The work of a chronic typhoid germ distributor. *JAMA*. 1907;48(24):2019–2022.

14. Ellis Island in 1905. Washington, DC: Library of Congress, Prints and Photographs Division: LC-USZ62-37784.

15. Bateman-House A, Fairchild A. Medical examination of immigrants at Ellis Island. *Virtual Mentor*. 2008;10(4):235–241.

16. The Statue of Liberty, Ellis Island Foundation. Ellis Island History. 2016. Available at: http://www.libertyellisfoundation.org/ellis-island-history#1965. Accessed June 15, 2016.

17. Regulations to Control Communicable Diseases, 42 USC §264. Available at: https://www.law.cornell.edu/uscode/text/42/264. Accessed September 6, 2014.

18. Obama B. Executive Order—Revised list of quarantinable communicable diseases. 2014. Available at: https://www.whitehouse.gov/the-press-office/2014/07/31/executive-order-revised-list-quarantinable-communicable-diseases. Accessed September 5, 2014.

19. O'Donnell K. NJ Gov. Chris Christie to Ebola quarantine nurse: go ahead, sue me. NBC News. October 28, 2014. Available at: http://www.nbcnews.com/storyline/ebola-virus-outbreak/nj-gov-chris-christie-ebola-quarantine-nurse-go-ahead-sue-n235436. Accessed September 5, 2016.

20. National Humanities Center. The paper war over smallpox vaccination in Boston, 1721. Available at: http://nationalhumanitiescenter.org/pds/becomingamer/ideas/text5/smallpoxvaccination.pdf. Accessed March 3, 2017.

21. Boylston Z. *An Historical Account of the Small-Pox Inoculated in New England*. 2nd ed. Boston, MA: S. Gerrish and T. Hancock, Booksellers; 1730.

22. Adams J. Letter from John Adams to Abigail Adams, 26 June 1776. Adams Family Papers. June 26, 1776. Massachusetts Historical Society. Available at: http://www.masshist.org/digitaladams/archive/doc?id=L17760626ja. Accessed March 3, 2017.

23. Filsinger AL, Dwek R. George Washington and the first mass military inoculation. Library of Congress Science Reference Services. Available at: https://www.loc.gov/rr/scitech/GW&smallpoxinoculation.html. Accessed June 15, 2016.

24. Centers for Disease Control and Prevention. Measles (rubeola) cases and outbreaks. 2015. Available at: http://www.cdc.gov/measles/cases-outbreaks.html. Accessed May 16, 2016.

25. Sydenstricker E. The incidence of influenza among persons of different economic status during the epidemic of 1918. *Public Health Rep*. 1931;46(4):154–170.

26. Schneider D, Lilienfeld DE. *Lilienfeld's Foundations of Epidemiology*. New York, NY: Oxford University Press; 2015.

27. Centers for Disease Control and Prevention. Syndromic surveillance for bioterrorism following the attacks on the World Trade Center—New York City, 2001. *MMWR Morb Mortal Wkly Rep*. 2002;51(spec no):13–15.

28. Syndromic surveillance data submission. 2014. Available at: https://www.healthit.gov/providers-professionals/achieve-meaningful-use/menu-measures/syndromic-surveillance-data-submission. Accessed May 17, 2016.

29. May L, Chretien J-P, Pavlin JA. Beyond traditional surveillance: applying syndromic surveillance to developing settings—opportunities and challenges. *BMC Public Health*. 2009;9:242.

30. Fall AG, Diaïté A, Seck MT, et al. West Nile virus transmission in sentinel chickens and potential mosquito vectors, Senegal River Delta, 2008–2009. *Int J Environ Res Public Health*. 2013;10(10):4718–4727.

31. Chaskopoulou A, Dovas CI, Chaintoutis SC, et al. Detection and early warning of West Nile virus circulation in Central Macedonia, Greece, using sentinel chickens and mosquitoes. *Vector Borne Zoonotic Dis*. 2013;13(10):723–732.

32. Healy JM, Reisen WK, Kramer VL, et al. Comparison of the efficiency and cost of West Nile virus surveillance methods in California. *Vector Borne Zoonotic Dis*. 2015;15(2):147–155.

33. Schurer JM, Hill JE, Fernando C, Jenkins EJ. Sentinel surveillance for zoonotic parasites in companion animals in indigenous communities of Saskatchewan. *Am J Trop Med Hyg*. 2012;87(3):495–498.

34. Faraji A, Unlu I. The eye of the tiger, the thrill of the fight: effective larval and adult control measures against the Asian tiger mosquito, *Aedes albopictus* (*Diptera: Culicidae*), in North America. *J Med Entomol*. 2016;53(3):1029–1047.35. World Health Organization. WHO Director-General summarizes the outcome of the Emergency Committee regarding clusters of microcephaly and Guillain-Barré syndrome. 2016. Available at: http://www.who.int/mediacentre/news/statements/2016/emergency-committee-zika-microcephaly/en. Accessed September 6, 2016.

36. Beck J. Should the Olympics be postponed because of Zika? *The Atlantic*. 2016. Available at: http://www.theatlantic.com/health/archive/2016/06/rio-de-janeiro-brazil-olympics-zika-risk-postpone-cancel-move/485183. Accessed September 6, 2016.

37. Fox M. Florida may have a second non-travel-related case of Zika. NBC News. July 21, 2016. Available at: http://www.nbcnews.com/storyline/zika-virus-outbreak/florida-may-have-second-non-travel-related-case-zika-n614481. Accessed September 5, 2016.

38. Verhage J, Silva S. Zika risks jeopardizing Florida's $90 billion tourism industry. *Bloomberg Markets*. August 22, 2016. Available at: http://www.bloomberg.com/news/articles/2016-08-22/zika-risks-jeopardizing-florida-s-90-billion-tourism-industry. Accessed September 6, 2016.

39. Carroll J, Gorgas WC, McCaw W, et al. *Yellow Fever: A Compilation of Various Publications: Results of the Work of Major Walter Reed, Medical Corps, and the Yellow Fever Commission*. Washington, DC: US Government Printing Office; 1911.

40. Centers for Disease Control and Prevention, Division of Vector-Borne Diseases. 2015. Available at: http://www.cdc.gov/ncezid/dvbd. Accessed September 5, 2016.

41. Robson M, Schneider D, Marentes C, Villanueva E. Field conditions for agricultural workers in the El Paso, Texas region. *New Solut*. 2001;11(2):141–148.

42. Gebbie K, Merrill J, Tilson HH. The public health workforce. *Health Aff (Millwood).* 2002;21(6):57–67.

43. US Department of Energy. Hanford Site. Available at: http://energy.gov/em/hanford-site. Accessed September 5, 2016.

44. US Environmental Protection Agency. The Love Canal tragedy. 1979. https://www.epa.gov/aboutepa/love-canal-tragedy. Accessed September 6, 2016.

45. US Environmental Protection Agency. EPA Superfund Program: A,L. Taylor (Valley of the Drums), Brooks, KY. Available at: https://cumulis.epa.gov/supercpad/cursites/csitinfo.cfm?id=0402072. Accessed September 6, 2016.

46. National Institutes of Health, US National Library of Medicine. TRI and Superfund Environmental Maps. TOXMAP. 2016. Available at: https://toxmap.nlm.nih.gov/toxmap/flex. Accessed March 3, 2017.

47. Nelson C, Lurie N, Wasserman J, Zakowski S, Leuschner KJ. *Conceptualizing and Defining Public Health Emergency Preparedness.* Santa Monica, CA: RAND Corporation; 2008.

48. Office of the Assistant Secretary for Preparedness and Response. National Health Security Strategy and Implementation Plan. Available at: http://www.phe.gov/Preparedness/planning/authority/nhss/Pages/strategy.aspx. Accessed September 6, 2016.

49. *Public Health Preparedness Capabilities: National Standards for State and Local Planning.* Washington, DC: Centers for Disease Control and Prevention; 2011.

50. American Public Health Association. Advocacy for public health. Available at: https://www.apha.org/policies-and-advocacy/advocacy-for-public-health. Accessed June 10, 2016.

51. National Association of County and City Health Officials . Policy and advocacy. Available at: http://www.naccho.org/advocacy. Accessed June 10, 2016.

52. Society of Public Health Educators. SOPHE's advocacy. Available at: http://www.sophe.org/advocacy.cfm. Accessed June 10, 2016.

53. Healthy People 2020. Disparities user guide. Available at: https://www.healthypeople.gov/2020/disparities-user-guide. Accessed September 7, 2016.

54. American Public Health Association. Health equity. Available at: https://www.apha.org/topics-and-issues/health-equity. Accessed September 7, 2016.

55. Robert Wood Johnson Foundation. Shaking up systems to achieve health equity. 2016. Available at: http://www.rwjf.org/en/culture-of-health/2016/03/shaking-up-systems.html. Accessed September 7, 2016.

II. TOOLS AND CASE STUDIES

4

OVERVIEW OF TOOLS AND CASE STUDIES

Selected tools used by public health and planning professionals, as well as case studies highlighting their use, are presented in Chapters 5 through 10. This chapter serves as a quick reference, offering brief summaries of each tool and data about each case.

Tools

In this chapter you will find the 18 tools presented in this book in alphabetical order, along with the chapter in which each tool is highlighted. The listings following the name of each tool provide (1) information on the definition and type of tool, (2) an explanation about how extensively the tool is used, and (3) any prerequisites to the tool's use.

Accessing and Interpreting Population Data (Chapter 6)

1. Accessing and analyzing demographic information at the county, local government, census tract, and block levels to find age, race/ethnicity, socioeconomic status, and other demographic patterns that can help inform decisions to protect human health and the environment.
2. Almost universal use of data in public health and planning; sophistication of analysis varies.
3. Already prepared data can be easily downloaded with only limited preparation. More demanding analyses require gathering, weighting, and then analyzing raw data. Expert help is advised for more complex applications.

Building and Zoning Codes (Chapter 10)

1. Legal requirements administered at the local scale that control what can be located at a site and how it is to be designed and operated to provide at least minimal protection to users and nearby stakeholders.

2. Have existed for centuries and in some places the requirements have been replaced by more performance-based codes.
3. A combination of efforts by attorneys, land-use planners, architects, and public health officials.

Checklists (Chapter 5)

1. An ordered list of concerns and actions to be periodically scanned to make sure that every issue is at least considered.
2. Widely used for keeping track of complex multiple-stage projects.
3. An experienced manager will be able to most effectively construct and use checklists to oversee and direct specific projects and avoid obvious mistakes, such as failure to coordinate with other managers at key times.

Collaborative Problem Solving (Chapter 8)

1. A multistage process involving a relatively small group of key participants who work together to arrive at a decision about a specific project or program on behalf of parties who are responsible for the project or program.
2. Used only when there are sufficient resources and time to consider many options with major long-term implications.
3. Group leader must be trained, objective, and respected and have resources to build and maintain a strong group and technical support staff.

Benefit and Cost Analysis (Chapter 9)

1. A set of analytical methods that are used to calculate and compare the lifecycle economic benefits and costs of a set of projects or programs.
2. Widely used to support capital investment and complex infrastructure programs and many other public and private programs.
3. Strong background in economics is essential.

Environmental Impact Statements (Chapter 9)

1. An ordered set of analyses and interactions required by federal and some state and local governments to assess the environmental consequences of projects or programs.

2. Required by the National Environmental Policy Act of 1970 of all major federally supported projects and those that require federal permits, licenses, and other legal approvals.
3. Multidisciplinary teams of experts in physical and social sciences required to gather, assess, and integrate data-based findings and advise decision-makers about a preferred option, a no-action alternative, and other options.

Environmental Justice Analysis (Chapter 7)

1. A process for measuring and determining the extent to which a population that has been legally identified as disadvantaged is impacted by a policy and is able to provide their input about that policy.
2. Required after Executive Order 12898 in 1994 in the United States; increased use as a result of environmental impact statement requirements.
3. Requires understanding of the political, social, and economic consequences, as well as the human health and environmental consequences, of proposed projects and plans and ability to use health impact analysis, environmental impact assessment, risk analysis, population, and other data sets and tools to address impacts on environmental justice populations.

Green Building Practices and Sustainable Development (Chapter 10)

1. Processes for building and using the environment in ways that are more protective of human health, safety, and ecological systems both for current and future generations.
2. Increasing trend in many places across the globe, especially as applied to land use planning, the building and operations of indoor environments, and the building envelope.
3. Requires the ability to use resources more efficiently and protectively and to understand the economic consequences of building choices in specific locations throughout the lifecycle of a land use.

Hazard Mitigation Analysis (Chapter 6)

1. A federally mandated planning process that requires states and many local governments to determine what and where hazards exist and what steps can be

taken to eliminate or at least reduce the likelihood of the event occurring and the consequences.

2. A relatively new mandate required if a major event occurs and the state seeks support from the Federal Emergency Management Agency. Communities were involved in mitigation before the legal requirement, but the requirement clearly places the key responsibility for integrating basic planning, environmental health, and hazard management at the local- and small-region scales.

3. Multidisciplinary teams with training and experience in hazards, risk, mitigation, and resilience are essential to guide state, regional, and especially local-scale planning.

Health Impact Assessment (Chapter 5)

1. An ordered process to examine human health and safety impacts of small and medium-sized projects and programs and to suggest solutions to reduce risk.

2. Major increase in use during the past decade to analyze policy options in transportation, recreation, and rebuilding neighborhoods, among others.

3. Formal training by an experienced health impact assessment expert is essential.

Indoor Air Quality (Chapter 10)

1. A set of checklists, mathematical models, design, and engineered design features that reduce public exposure to airborne hazards that may be biological, chemical, and physical in origin.

2. The need for such tools has expanded because people spend 90 percent or more of their time indoors and can be subjected to unacceptable exposures that are more hazardous than those found outside.

3. Awareness and need have increased but more expertise is needed to make decisions that will reduce exposures.

Planning and Design Charrettes (Chapter 8)

1. Design options built with physical books or computers to help stakeholders understand what a specific design option would look like and then to solicit stakeholder input on the options.

2. Used when multiple options are plausible, time is available, and stakeholder input is essential.

3. Strong design and communications skills are a must.

Public Information Gathering and Outreach (Chapter 5)

1. Surveys, focus groups, public meetings, Web sites, and other tools that allow decision-makers to provide information to stakeholders and obtain information from them.
2. Widely used by decision-makers in public policy formation to inform parties and themselves about public values, perceptions, and preferences.
3. Each of these tools has unique requirements, which means that multiple experts must work together.

Mapping as a Way of Communicating Information (Chapter 6)

1. Drawing maps at different scales that reveal important spatial attributes of projects and programs to help decision-makers and other interested parties better understand implications.
2. Massive use following the development of high-speed computers and mapping software.
3. Novices can draw simple maps, but complex ones require experienced cartographers.

Political Process Assessment (Chapter 7)

1. Process that tracks the building of political pressure to change government and private policy and practice.
2. Rarely used proactively, rather observed after the pressure has reached a high level and action is needed to improve conditions.
3. Requires experts who understand the issue, its historical roots, and political underpinnings, which typically means individuals with training in political science, law, and public policy.

Regional Economic Impact Analysis (Chapter 9)

1. Quantitative analytical tools used to estimate direct, indirect, and induced economic impacts of projects or programs over time by business sector and across places.
2. Used when economic impacts are sufficiently important and nuanced to estimate economic impacts for decision-makers.
3. Strength in quantitative economic modeling is essential.

Risk Analysis (Chapter 8)

1. A set of process and analytical tools used to determine what risks can occur, their likelihood, consequences, and how consequences can be prevented or reduced in magnitude and responded to in order to promote recovery.
2. Primary use is to reduce risk to human health and the environment from biological, chemical, and physical hazards.
3. Multidisciplinary expertise from bench science to risk communications is required.

Social Network Analysis (Chapter 7)

1. Quantitative and qualitative tools and processes used to provide analysts with insights about key players who create, expand, and otherwise manage decision-making programs.
2. Rapid expansion of capability with Web-based communications that are complementing and in some cases exceeding face-to-face contacts as sources of information and policy ideas.
3. Probes of key players and organizations are feasible with limited training. More detailed understanding requires training in the use of computer packages.

Case Studies

The tools listed previously are illustrated with case studies across seven U.S. states (Table 4.1). These case studies were selected primarily because the authors were familiar with their challenges and outcomes and had ready access to information about them that could demonstrate the value of using the tools. The selected case studies also represent a variety of settings across the United States, many of which may be useful for planners, public health workers, and policymakers alike.

Final Thoughts

Chapters 5 through 10 are roughly split between the presentation of tools and case studies that demonstrate how these tools were used in real situations. The chapters begin by assuming an issue has arisen that you and/or colleagues need to address. We then list three tools that might be used, describing each in detail so you can decide how they might work in the hypothetical case. Next, one or more case studies are presented to illustrate how the tools were used to address actual problems. Not every tool was successfully used in every case study and, when they were not used, we explain why. Each chapter offers final thoughts about the issues and tools discussed, followed by references.

Table 4.1. Summary Information About Eleven Case Studies

Case Study	Chapter	Site Description	County, State	Comments
Middlesex Greenway	5	Older suburbs	Middlesex, New Jersey	Former rail line turned into recreation area
Bloomfield Avenue traffic calming	5	Older suburbs	Essex, New Jersey	Traffic calming of a heavily used road artery
Texas hazard mitigation	6			Hazard mitigation planning
• State		All 254 counties	• State of Texas	
• Houston-Galveston		Large metro region	• 80+ local governments in southeast Texas	
• Galveston City		City of ~50,000 on a barrier island in the Gulf of Mexico	• Galveston County, Texas	
California's food security program	7	Central city	Los Angeles, California	Efforts to improve food security and nutrition in a poor community
San Diego Veterans Village	7	Mixed-use area in major city	San Diego, California	Multiple programs to assist war veterans
Fernald nuclear weapon site	8	Mixed urban and rural area in Cincinnati region	Hamilton and Butler, Ohio	Remediation of former nuclear weapons material refining site
Denver International Airport	9	Eastern edge of Denver metro region	10-county metro region, Colorado	New airport and extensions
Sparrows Point Liquefied Natural Gas Application	9	Small community at eastern edge of Baltimore County	Baltimore County, Maryland	Proposed liquefied natural gas import terminal site
Green building in New Orleans Post-Katrina	10	A housing development and school in formerly devastated areas of the City of New Orleans	Orleans Parish, Louisiana	Green building projects in two poor neighborhoods near the Mississippi River

5

ENHANCING A GOOD IDEA

Someone has just called your office to let you know that the federal government wants to turn over abandoned surplus land in your town for redevelopment. The town could use a new park site and a location for a school. Should you accept the gift? If so, under what conditions? This chapter begins by describing checklists and a set of public information gathering and communications tools. These tools may be applied to almost every issue that comes before local health and planning departments, such as building a public swimming pool or a bicycle path; expanding park space; adding a garden, a zoo, or a health center; and so many other projects that should be win–win ones for a community. These same tools may be applied to more difficult challenges that are addressed later in this book, including brownfield cleanups and redevelopments, as well as the construction of new factories or transportation facilities. The third tool featured in this chapter is the health impact assessment (HIA), an important tool that is increasingly applied to a wide set of issues. The chapter uses case studies of a greenway on a former railroad line and a proposed traffic-calming project to illustrate the use of the following tools:

- Checklists
- Public information gathering and outreach (surveys, focus groups, public meetings, newsletters, Web sites, etc.)
- Health impact assessment

Checklists

A checklist provides a simple review of issues that should be considered to differentiate a good idea from a not-so-good one. The first author began to develop a checklist four decades ago when asked by a community to assess a project proposed in a floodplain. The original checklist had five questions, has been modified multiple times, and the one displayed here has 18 primary and 49 secondary questions (Table 5.1). The questions directly relate to human health, safety, and mental health. They cover six topics: air quality, fresh water, waste management, ecology and sustainability, sensitive human populations, and social and economic issues related to mental health. Each topic starts with a primary probe, and if the answer to that question is "yes," then further investigation is warranted.[1,3]

Table 5.1. Human Health–Oriented Checklist Questions

Air Quality Issues

1. Will the discharges into the atmosphere—those coming directly from a commercial facility, housing development, transportation project, road construction, remediation and restoration, recreation, or other type of project (hereafter referred to as "the project")—be different in quality from the current conditions of the ambient environment, and/or will the project notably change the quantity of emissions in the area?
   1.1. Will the emissions lead to a violation of a national ambient air quality standard(s) or exacerbate an existing violation?
   1.2. Will the discharge include toxic organic or inorganic substances?

2. Will traffic in and out of the project (from workers, residents, recreationists, shoppers, and others) produce serious traffic congestion?
   2.1. Will emissions lead to localized violations of national ambient air quality standards, for example, carbon monoxide and fine particulates?
   2.2. Will this traffic congestion be near a residential area, school, place of worship, or other site with sensitive receptors?
   2.3. Will the risk to bicycle riders and/or walkers be increased as a result of the project?

3. Will construction related to the project, and subsequently its operation, and attendant transportation activities produce a noise level above the ambient?
   3.1. Will the level exceed 55 dB(A) outdoors or 45 dB(A) inside a residential or public facility, school, hospital, recreation, or shopping area?
   3.2. Will this level ever exceed 80 dB(A) during the day or 70 dB(A) during the night?

4. Will the project and related activities produce an odor?
   4.1. Will the odor be apparent in a residential neighborhood, shopping, recreation, or other sensitive area?

5. Will the activity require a stack, call for any other prominent vertical structure, or produce visible emissions?
   5.1. Will these be visible more than one-half mile away?

Fresh Water Resource Issues

6. Will the project produce a process discharge or runoff discharge that will be directed to a local stream used for drinking water or fishing? To a local groundwater source?
   6.1. Will the discharge threaten a drinking water quality standard?
   6.2. Will the discharge enter the water body at levels above the ambient and change the water salinity, pH, or oxygen levels, or will it contain toxins or biological agents?
   6.3. Will the discharge discolor the water or contribute to eutrophication?
   6.4. Will recreational fishing activities be threatened?
   6.5. Will the project require redirecting or channeling a water body?

7. Will the project produce a discharge into a salt water body?
   7.1. Will a valuable ecosystem be compromised and/or will waterborne recreational activities be threatened?
   7.2. Will the temperature of the salt water body be affected by the discharge?

8. Will additional impervious cover be required for the activity?
   8.1. Will the impervious cover impact a nearby surface and/or underground supply?
   8.2. Will the quality of the discharge threaten the quality of the water?
   8.3. Will the project contain green roofs and/or retention basins?
   8.4. What is the plan to maintain these engineered systems?

(Continued)

Table 5.1. (Continued)

Waste Management Issues: Solid and Liquid Elements

9. Will solid and semi-liquid waste from the project be different from residential waste?
   9.1. Are these wastes degradable in the environment? Over what period of time?
   9.2. Is any of this waste toxic, flammable, carcinogenic, or in other ways hazardous?
   9.3. Will any waste be stored on site? If so, how will it be managed to prevent exposures through water supplies and direct human contact?

10. Will waste be transported off site?
   10.1. Will the vehicles (trains, trucks) increase congestion, lead to higher noise or odor levels, and possibly be a threat to human health and safety?
   10.2. Assuming that some of the waste is hazardous, what provisions are in place to protect nearby populations against accidents or deliberate attacks aimed at spreading the waste?

Ecological and Sustainability Issues

11. Will the project sit on a hilly or ecologically sensitive land?
   11.1. Will the soils and bedrock easily erode?
   11.2. Will all or any of the projects be located in the 100-year floodplain? An area that has had mudslides, earthquakes, or other natural hazard events?
   11.3. Will species be reduced or eliminated? Are any of these protected by federal or state statute?
   11.4. What plans exist to remediate any ecological issues?
   11.5. Will the project reuse existing building or waste products, including water; have solar or other renewable energy sources; or in other ways demonstrate a commitment to more sustainable and resilient building and operating practices?

Issues Involving Sensitive Human Populations

12. Is the resident population near the facility disproportionately poor, black, Latino, or Native American?
   12.1. Is there empirical evidence that this area already has a disproportionate burden of unwanted land uses?
   12.2. Is there likely to be an environmental justice challenge raised?

13. Is there a nearby hospital, school, or facility that houses disabled, seniors, and other individuals with health issues?
   13.1. Is this facility equipped and is its management able to cope with development of the area?
   13.2. Is this facility able to respond to events that might be triggered by transportation issues related to the project facility?

14. Will the facility cause undesirable animals to move to nearby areas?
   14.1. Will rats, mice, deer, predators, or other undesirable species migrate to nearby residential areas?
   14.2. What plans exist to manage issues related to undesirable animals?

Social and Economic Issues Related to Mental Health

15. Will the project impact nearby land uses?
   15.1. Is the project incompatible with existing land uses, thereby potentially leading to human health and safety concerns?
   15.2. Will the project threaten property values?
   15.3. Will the project block scenic views or be visible from recreation areas?
   15.4. Will the project detract from culturally significant sites?
   15.5. Will existing water, sewer, electrical, computer-related, and other systems in the vicinity of the project's site need to be replaced or increased and thereby impact these areas with noise, odors, and other undesirable effects?

(Continued)

Table 5.1. (Continued)

16.	Will the project change public service requirements in the community?
	16.1. Will new police, fire, garbage collection, schools, and other services be required?
	16.2. Are the current fire and police departments able to manage any fire or hazardous substance release from the project?
	16.3. How will upgrades of current service be funded?
17.	Will jobs change in the area as a result of the project?
	17.1. Will the project increase or decrease job opportunities for nearby residents?
	17.2. What kinds of jobs would be created or lost? What level of education will be required for new jobs?
	17.3. Will the project threaten existing local retailing and service jobs?
	17.4. Does the area have a plan to supply job training as needed?
18.	Will the project notably change the fiscal base of the community?
	18.1. Will more tax-paying entities be created or enhanced by the project, or will they be lost?
	18.2. Will there be an agreement to hire a people who live in the surrounding area?

Source: Based on Greenberg et al. (1979)[1] and Greenberg and Weiner (2014).[2]

We regard checklists as living documents to be modified as knowledge expands and issues change. As their purpose is to make sure that a key issue is not missed, checklists can be employed to target specific users' needs. For example, the first author and colleagues prepared a checklist of more than 250 items for the U.S. Department of Energy with regard to selecting sustainable nuclear waste management practices at its former nuclear weapons sites.[4] Checklists were also used in the two case studies in this chapter to determine if a project was suitable for an HIA.

Public Information Gathering and Outreach

Decision-makers, experts, and advocates need information about public preferences, values, and perceptions. They also need platforms to communicate with the public. Those who fail to understand or who choose to ignore the public before embarking on a project, or those who fail to communicate their progress or failures along the way, are following a path that will likely lead to serious public rebuke. Surveys, focus groups, public meetings, and other outreach tools allow those planning, implementing, and evaluating projects to get important public input.

Surveys

Surveys are a common tool for gathering information. The number one problem with surveys is that many of the questions are formatted in such a way that respondents do not understand them. Thus, short, simple questions in language that everyone can understand, without professional jargon, are advised. It is vital to pretest questions with representatives of the intended audience before using them. We suggest avoiding reinventing the wheel and instead reusing already-published questions that have a track record.

Overly long surveys can undermine the objective of gathering information. We were recently asked to review a survey that was to be filled out by senior citizens. The questions were well written, but it took us 35 minutes to fill out was supposed to be a 10-minute survey. A simple survey might take 10 to 15 minutes, but the maximum should be 20 minutes because respondent fatigue sets in. At that point, people become impatient and either refuse to answer questions or do not think seriously about their answers.

Surveys done over the telephone need to be done not only during the day but also in the evening and on weekends. Avoiding holidays is a good idea, as is not surveying after a major national event because many potential respondents are not available and/or are too distracted to reliably participate. When population-based sampling is done over the phone, respondents should include both landline and cell phone users. Unless a large proportion of cell phone users are contacted and respond, survey results will be biased toward older community members who do not rely exclusively on cell phones. Unfortunately, cell phone samples are much more expensive than landline ones because cell phone users move and take their numbers with them. It may take many calls to find even a single person who is eligible to respond to the survey. Our current experience is that we need to contact a number 8 to 10 times to obtain a response rate of 20 to 25 percent.[2] We warn that phone surveys are a serious investment, and we have paid on average $100,000 to obtain 1,200 to 1,500 valid responses.

Mail surveys, like phone surveys, have limitations. Even when the survey includes a self-addressed, stamped return envelope, a good response rate can no longer be assumed. This has led some researchers to use "mail-push-to-Web," in which a postal mailing effort directs potential respondents to a survey Web site. With the increasing use of Internet surveys over the past decade, many people respond on a smartphone, "pad" computers, and other handheld electronic communication devices.[2] Those responsible for survey design and implementation should be cognizant of how the questions and answer choices will appear on the screens of various types of electronic devices.

Regardless of the methods used to elicit information, survey scales should be consistent so readers or listeners do not have to readjust their thinking and make mistakes in responding. If a large group of potential respondents do not speak English, it is important for someone to be standing by who can ask the questions in other languages.

Random sampling is the gold standard for gathering population survey data, whether done through the mail, via landline and cell phone, or by using a Web site or social media. The goal of random sampling is to make sure that everyone in the group of interest has an equal chance of being contacted.[5-8] However, if resources are limited and time is short, convenience samples are the obvious choice for obtaining information from the public. This means talking to people at or after a public meeting, or in a park, store, or other public gathering place. The questions are normally answered on paper, taken home and mailed in, or answered on the Web. Convenience samples have the advantage of gathering data quickly and inexpensively, but they may not be representative of the larger population and thus may yield misleading results.

How important is it for the data to be representative of the target population? Very! For instance, if you were doing a survey to collect data about senior citizen needs in an area, using landline phones might work. However, the same would not be true if the issue of concern was about developing plans for a park for teenage bike riders. In other words, the collection mode needs to be fitted to the population of interest.

How large should a sample be? The answer depends upon how much confidence you want to have in your results. Suppose someone did a random sample survey using 200 respondents and found that the proportion favoring construction of a new park was 54 percent. The 95 percent confidence limits around those results are about 6.9 percent. This means that if the survey was repeated using the same sample size of 200, 95 percent of the time it would yield between 47.1 and 60.9 percent of respondents supporting the project. If the sample size was 400, the interval would shrink to between 49.1 and 58.9 percent; at 600 it would be between 50 and 58 percent. In short, it takes a relatively large sample to be certain, which is why large samples are taken before an important election. Once a random sample exceeds 800, the confidence interval no longer shrinks much, and spending additional resources to increase the sample size may not be justified. Of course, people's responses are not always truthful. They sometimes tell the interviewer what they think the interviewer wants to hear, and they may not be truthful when honest responses reveal a potential bias that they do not want the interviewer to know about.

The choice of a random or convenience sample framework, the number and order of questions, and the mode of collection require expert consultation and heavily depend upon the budget for the project. Almost every major university will have several experts who have conducted many surveys. They are likely to have knowledge about banks of questions that have already been tested and validated and should have experience with phone, mail, and Internet surveys. Some researchers find it helps to pay respondents for their time to get a higher response rate, but this will depend upon the project budget.

Focus Groups

Not every project proposed has a budget, sufficient time before launch, or even requirements for collecting quantitative data from a target population. One or more focus groups might provide sufficient information to steer a project toward success. A focus group is a low-cost tool in which a facilitator guides a group of people though a set of questions designed to elicit their preferences, values, perceptions, and other issues related to the project. We have used focus groups to identify the key questions we should ask before launching a survey, and we have employed focus groups after a survey to shed further light on our results. The idea is to engage people in a guided conversation and to obtain important insights.

Two critical issues for focus groups are the choice of the facilitator (moderator) and group membership. Subject matter experts are not usually good facilitators for several reasons. First, dealing with people in an open forum is not an easy thing to do and most experts have not developed this skill. Second, experts may have biases. Even if they do not, the group members may perceive them as being biased. Hence, it is strongly recommended that the moderator have no real stake in the outcome. The second critical issue is setting criteria for focus group membership. We strongly recommend that people be grouped by obvious criteria such as age and location.[9,10] For example, a new park might warrant a focus group of seniors who live near the proposed site. Another group might be people who live farther from the proposed park but who might use it for very different reasons or at different times. Group membership should not include those who are ideologically committed to or against a proposed project because they likely will try to dominate the conversation. When this happens, other group members may mentally disengage or even leave the group. A good focus group features interchanges among the members, but it may not necessarily lead to consensus. What the results will provide are helpful insights.

Most public health and planning officials know people who could be part of a productive and constructive focus group and they should be encouraged to make membership recommendations. For context, it would be typical to hold three to five focus group meetings on ideas for a new park. After the meetings are completed, the results should be interpreted and difficult issues resolved. There are many forms of focus groups, and we again suggest that most universities have faculty with many years of experience in eliciting public information. It is likely they would be willing to help with focus groups.

Public Meetings and Other Outreach Tools

Public meetings are part of the democratic process and some are even required by law. It is likely that every reader of this book has attended at least one public meeting where all attendees were given an opportunity to voice their views.[11-13] Occasionally, public meetings can get out of control, particularly when those with strong preferences and ideologies try to preclude others from speaking. Sometimes the audience may become angry because they perceive that a decision has already been made and the meeting is just a rubber stamp to fulfill legal requirements. However, there is another side of public meetings. Attendees can be informed about a project, be asked to fill out surveys, join focus groups, join teams that are forming to examine elements of a project, express their views, and provide documents to the meeting organizers. It is fair to say that all of the above may happen when members of the public feel strongly about a subject. If they are apathetic, they may simply not attend. When it comes to a new project, a slightly rowdy crowd at a public meeting might be better than none at all.

Increasingly, the Web is emerging as an option for reaching those who have neither the time nor the inclination to attend public meetings. Project sponsors, citizen advisory groups appointed to represent a community, and/or other parties can post meeting times and locations, fact sheets, minutes from prior meetings, opportunities for participation, and other information. Project-based Web sites may also provide an opportunity for people to post questions and information. Establishing a special phone number for people to call in, pick up information, and ask questions about a new project is another option. If either a Web or landline opportunity to engage the public is established, it is imperative that responses are provided to queries within a day or two. If people are given a chance to ask questions, those questions need to be answered in a timely fashion. If not, the result will be a hostile public, a reality we know from being yelled at by people who expected immediate callbacks.

The last set of options for public outreach is providing information about projects to local radio and television stations, as well as the print media. Depending upon the region, we have seen other public outreach strategies employed. For instance, we have seen storefronts in strategic locations that offer residents an opportunity to walk in, pick up information, and speak with project staff. We have seen project managers establish a physical presence in the community by sending knowledgeable speakers to schools, community meetings, and other public gathering places such as county fairs. We have been speakers at several of these and have been involved in outreach programs in remote rural areas as well as in city neighborhoods. We know there is no formula for picking outreach tools.[14] The most effective outreach tools should be selected in concert with local media experts and community representatives.

Health Impact Assessment

An HIA combines a compact process with a set of analytical tools to assess the human health impacts of a proposed project, plan, or action. In many ways, the objectives of an HIA are similar to those of an environmental impact statement (EIS). Both seek to evaluate a planned action; both have a scoping phase, data gathering and evaluation phases, and public participation phases. There are, however, several marked differences.[3,15,16] Perhaps the most important of these is that the EIS process has been required for federal projects under the National Environmental Policy Act since 1970. While they deal with public health impacts, EISs typically cover ecological concerns rather than economic and social ones. They often require massive data gathering and simulation analyses. As a

Table 5.2. Steps in a Typical Health Risk Assessment

Step	Question Addressed
1. Screening	Does the project/action warrant a health impact assessment?
2. Scoping	What human health impacts should be the focus?
3. Analysis of impacts	What are the type, likelihood, and magnitude of the negative and positive impacts?
4. Managing impacts	What are recommendations for reducing negative health impacts and increasing positive ones?
5. Communications	How are the results going to be presented?
6. Follow-up	How are the results going to be monitored?

result, EISs are long—typically 1,000 or more pages—and they include shorter environmental assessments (EAs) that might be between 100 and 300 pages. There are between 250 and 500 EISs done every year and thousands of EAs (see Chapter 9).

In contrast to EISs, HIAs are primarily voluntary, although this might change in the future. They are narrowly directed toward local projects with public health implications. HIAs typically use existing data, although surveys and other limited data-gathering efforts can take place. They also concentrate on decisions that clearly can be influenced by their results. Thus, HIAs fill an important gap in the public health and planning toolbox. They assess the need for a project, but not to the extent of a community health needs assessment that considers the full range of community needs. They assess human health and safety risks, but not to the extent of risk assessment, which will include considerable data gathering, simulation modeling, and engineering. The great strength of the HIA is that it fits a niche at the local–small region scale. HIAs tend to involve communities at a very early stage, typically in a six-step process (Table 5.2).

HIAs have several levels. The desk-based process typically takes place over a few weeks and leads to an overview of the potential impacts of a proposed project. A second, intermediate level typically takes over a few months and provides more detail on potential impacts. A comprehensive HIA may take six months or longer and provides more information for each of the six steps listed in Table 5.2. Although HIAs typically are used for prospective analysis, it is possible to do retrospective ones.

Organizations supporting the use of HIAs include governmental agencies such as the U.S. Centers for Disease Control and Prevention and regional powers such as the European Union, as well as nations such as Australia, Canada, New Zealand, and Thailand, among others. The Web sites of the World Health Organization, the World Bank, the National Association of County and City Health Officials, Pew Charitable Trusts, and many other organizations encourage participation in, provide funds for, and in many other ways promote the use of HIAs. Indeed, the reach of this tool has figuratively exploded. For instance, there are innumerable journal articles related to HIAs during the past decade, recent texts,[17–20] and ongoing informational Web sites and blogs[21-23] on the topic. Many agencies and professional organizations provide a variety of HIA training courses—from free, short online courses[24] to in-depth multiday trainings.[25] Our technical staff was trained by experts from the Pew Charitable Trust, and now other organizations are offering training. We recommend that those performing HIAs obtain certification, as it will raise the credibility of their results.

Case Studies

New Jersey is the most densely populated state and has the road traffic density to match its population. As measured by ethnic/racial diversity and foreign-born population, New Jersey is, along with California and New York, one of the most diverse states in the nation. Because it once served as a major manufacturing center, New Jersey has many industrial and transportation sites that have long since been abandoned. We offer two HIA applications that highlight these major features of the state.

Middlesex Greenway Access Plan

During the heyday of the U.S. industrial era, manufacturing was the major source of jobs. Trains carried raw materials and manufactured products across the country and, even today, rail remains a critically important and extremely efficient means of transportation.[26] However, many rail lines have become expendable. One of these rail lines ran through the central New Jersey towns of Metuchen, Edison, and Woodbridge. The Lehigh Valley Railroad shipped coal from Pennsylvania to New Jersey and New York along this line. With the decline in the coal industry, the line was abandoned and the rail corridor was taken over by Middlesex County, an urban county with a population of 810,000. The county turned the abandoned corridor into a 3.5-mile-long greenway from Metuchen in the west to Woodbridge in the east. The center of the Greenway is 35 miles away from the Empire State Building and 41.2 miles from Trenton, the capital of New Jersey (about 35 minutes by mass transit and an hour by car).

The Middlesex Greenway, opened in 2012, is an approximately 10-foot-wide paved path through a mostly wooded corridor that should be attractive for walkers, joggers, and bikers. The first author took his two youngest grandchildren (1 and 2 years old) who ran and walked along the greenway for an hour on a summer day tossing stones, picking up twigs, and waving to passersby). It is intended to eventually become part of an East Coast Greenway that will run more than 1,000 miles between Key West, Florida, and southern Canada. The path is paved and runs through a complex environment, with new housing and landscaping sprouting up along the route in some places, while its rail heritage remains clear in others.

Despite the fact that the Middlesex Greenway is adjacent or close to parks, schools, senior citizens' residences and facilities and to various residential commercial, industrial, and institutional facilities, it is considered underutilized. In 2014, a group of university-based researchers,[27] government officials, not-for-profit groups, and residents came together to consider an HIA that would determine how increased use of this important resource would affect human health by the following actions:

- Increase physical activity.
- Decrease environmental exposures.
- Increase security along the path.
- Increase safety.
- Increase social cohesion.
- Improve the local economy.

Methods

All the tools described earlier in the chapter were used to develop the HIA. Given the population diversity along the Middlesex Greenway, considerable effort had to be devoted to engaging local residents and their representatives to discuss the project. These efforts included a large steering committee representing 15 organizations that attended up to four meetings to discuss key elements of increasing access to the greenway. Multiple open house events were held: two near the start of the project, one at a nearby senior citizen living facility, and one near the end of the project. Three roundtables were held to gain local input about safety, security, environmental health, physical activity, education and economic issues, and any other concerns.

The research team reviewed the black and gray literature, obtaining data from the following sources:

- U.S. Census Bureau (population attributes)
- Behavioral Risk Factor Surveillance System for New Jersey
- County health departments
- Local police reports
- Traffic incident reports
- Local professionals who had local data from recent studies

The researchers interviewed local health department staff, local medical staff from hospitals, and selected other experts. They conducted a convenience sample survey to obtain data about public awareness and utilization of the greenway and to learn about health and safety concerns. The survey had 40 questions, almost all with multiple parts. People were recruited at the initial open houses, through email solicitation, and from postings on organization Web sites. A total of 565 persons responded, mostly on a Web platform, but some through the distribution of paper surveys. The online survey was available in Spanish (7 percent of respondents were Hispanic).

At the HIA screening stage, the group used a checklist with 15 questions divided into questions about the value and need for an HIA, feasibility of conducting the HIA, and receptiveness of the decision-making process to an HIA. The evaluators and funders were looking for a pending decision with the following attributes:

- Decision could be enhanced with an HIA.
- Final decision about what was to be done had not been made.
- Sufficient time is available to inform the decision-making process.
- Stakeholders support the idea of an HIA.
- Decision-making process is open to HIA-based recommendations.

Results

The Middlesex Greenway has the potential to be a positive asset to public health because the area is so densely developed. Specifically, New Jersey is the only state with a population density exceeding 1,000 per square mile. A total of 213,000 people live in the three towns (3,705 people per square mile). The resource provides a rare location where nearby residents can jog, walk, stroll, bike, and contemplate without the sounds of urban traffic, other urban sounds, and disturbances.

The positive physical, mental, and social health effects of physical activity are documented in the literature. Physical activity reduces the likelihood of heart disease, stroke, diabetes, and high blood pressure. It reduces obesity and strengthens bones, muscles, and ligaments, all of which lead to physical and mental health benefits. Regular physical activity can reduce the likelihood of serious falls and the extent of fall-related injuries. Youth and every other age, not just seniors, benefit from regular exercise. Yet we know that most people are only willing to travel a short distance for physical activity, and they want to feel safe in the environment where they exercise.

The following opportunities and challenges were at the heart of the Middlesex Greenway project. Fifty-five percent of the population that responded to the survey self-identified as belonging to a racial or ethnic minority. Sixteen percent of the population residing within one-half mile of the greenway were 75 years of age or older, compared with 6 percent within one mile of it and 6 percent in the county as a whole. Eleven percent identified within one-half mile were disabled, compared with 8.7 percent and 8.3 percent in the one-mile radius surrounding it and within the county as a whole, respectively. This means that special arrangements should be made to institute traffic calming policies in the Middlesex Greenway area to permit more time to cross the street and to make sure that there are sidewalks along the streets and that the path itself is accessible to wheelchairs and walkers.

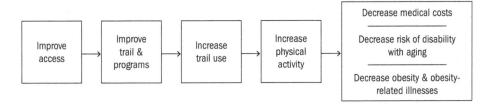

Source: Adapted from Lowrie et al. (2014).[27(p8)]

Figure 5.1. Causal Pathway Model, Middlesex Greenway

HIAs typically excel at producing results for different audiences. At the screening stage, there was sufficient interest and financial support provided to allow the researchers to perform an intermediate-level HIA over about a six-month period, which permitted detailed mapping and interpretation, surveying, and interviewing. The researchers drew one-half-mile and one-mile radii around the path. They found seven schools, parks, senior facilities, and local mass transit stops, as well as two farmer's markets, a YMCA, and other assets in the area. They identified some problems with access, including road-crossing issues and sidewalk problems.

Another strength of a typical HIA is that analysts are explicit about what causes various outcomes and who will benefit from the project or changes to the project. These points become valuable tools for discussion. We have reproduced one that focuses on the relationship between physical activity, obesity, and improved health outcomes (Figure 5.1). The diagram, in essence, diagrams the scientific rationale for the relationship among physical activity, obesity reduction, improved health, and lower medical costs. From left to right, improving access to the greenway, adding new programs, and increasing the use of the trail is expected to increase physical activity, which, in turn, reduces medical costs, the risk of disability with aging, and obesity. The latter is assumed to reduce the likelihood of obesity-related diseases. Readers of this book will already know that the real causal paths are more complicated. However, these kinds of charts help those who are not familiar with the background science.

Another way of interpreting the HIA for the Middlesex Greenway project is illustrated in Table 5.3, which summarizes the research team's findings about human health based on all of their work. For example, physical activity is expected to have positive impacts on public health, the probability is likely, and the impact level is considered to be high. The target groups are trail users, low-income people (particularly seniors) who do not have money to pay for health clubs, and the Hispanic population. As with the diagram in Figure 5.1, these findings are generalizations that do not fit every case, but they serve the purpose of focusing public attention on the key expected benefits.

Important insights were gained from the surveys, meetings, and interviews. With regard to the surveys, the data showed that college-educated, relatively affluent, and

Table 5.3. Summary of Findings From Middlesex Gateway Project

Health outcome	Direction	Likelihood	Impact	Impacted Population
Physical activity	+	Likely	High	Trail users, lower-income populations with limited access to paid health clubs, Hispanic population
Exposure to green space	+/−	Likely	Low	Trail users, children, people with allergies/asthma
Safety (crashes)	?	Uncertain	Medium	Trail users, drivers on area roads
Security (crime)	?	Unlikely	Medium	Trail users, nearby homes and businesses
Security (crime perception)	+	Possible	Medium	Trail users, senior citizens, women
Social interaction	+	Likely	High	Trail users, surrounding municipalities
Local economy	+	Possible	Low	Residents of surrounding municipalities

Source: Adapted from Lowrie et al. (2014).[27(p8)]

Note: + = may improve health; − = may detract from health; ? = unknown.

predominantly white women aged 31 to 64 years disproportionately were greenway users. Typically, they spent about 30 minutes on the path, but some spent one or two hours for exercise, mostly walking and biking. Metuchen residents, also predominantly white, disproportionately appeared to be users. The survey data also showed that two of the target groups, seniors and Hispanics, were not using the pathway as hoped and would need to be approached with outreach campaigns to engage them.

While acknowledging that the survey overrepresents middle-aged and relatively affluent women, 405 of the 565 respondents said they use the greenway. Almost one-quarter of them said that the presence of the Middlesex Greenway increased their level of physical activity by "a great deal," and another 45 percent said that it had increased it "somewhat." Almost 60 percent of nonusers said they would probably use it during the coming year. These are encouraging data.

Interesting and not surprising insights were gained about what would lead to more use of the greenway. Safety from crime, more accessible entry points, and special events were the priorities of more than one-fourth of the respondents, and between 10 and 24 percent wanted dedicated bicycle lanes, parking, benches, safer road crossings, exercise stations, and disability (Americans with Disabilities Act, or ADA) access. Interviews and meetings verified these data. The data also pointed to inadequate signage directing people to the Middlesex Greenway from population clusters, commercial areas, and transit stops, a point we experienced when it took us 20 minutes to find an entrance with parking nearby.

There was also interest in applying design principles to limit the likelihood of criminal activity along the greenway. Even though there might be air pollution from nearby auto sources along the path in several spots, this was not further explored because it was not a major concern of the participants and there were insufficient data.

Table 5.4. Recommendations From Middlesex Greenway Project

Enhance Usability and Expand Physical Fitness Options
• Improve access and use for bicycles. • Consider rental stations for bikes and in-line skates. • Provide benches and picnic tables in strategic locations. • Encourage use of activity loops for exercise. • Consider installing exercise stations in proximity to trail. • Facilitate connection between greenway and other parks and trails. • Provide signs indicating access for restrooms and refreshments.
Enhance Trail Cleanliness and Maintenance
• Install additional garbage and recycling cans, as well as dog refuse bags. • Install "no littering" signs. • Partner with local groups on cleanup programs, such as Adopt a Trail. • Facilitate easy ways to report graffiti.
Increase Use and Benefit by Vulnerable Subpopulations
• Involve local health providers to prescribe greenway use for weight reduction/health improvement. • Increase number of ADA-accessible ramps. • Implement chaperone program for seniors and disabled. • Increase access and awareness of greenway by NJ Transit bus riders. • Translate promotional and educational materials and signs, where appropriate, into Spanish. • Encourage safe use of greenway for school students.

Source: Adapted from Lowrie et al. (2014).[27(p66)]
Note: ADA = Americans with Disabilities Act.

Recommendations

The report offered 38 recommendations for physical activity, environmental exposures, security, safety, social cohesion, and the local economy. As space does not permit a full listing, we have reproduced only those for physical activity (Table 5.4). For instance, under enhancing usability and expanding physical fitness options, seven suggestions were provided that should make the Middlesex Greenway more accessible and appealing.

Each recommendation was accompanied by one or more strategies and actions to facilitate accomplishing the recommendation (not shown due to space constraints). For example, under "improve access and use for bicycles" the following actions were recommended:

- Improve/widen bike side-ramps with antiskid surfaces, where possible, alongside stairs.
- Provide/improve secure bicycle parking.
- Consider bike repair and air fill kiosks.
- Install new access ramps at strategic access points where feasible.

The strategic section of the HIA estimated how long each of these strategies would take to succeed and listed partners to work with to achieve them. The research team recognized the importance of communicating their results. They sent a draft of the HIA to the project steering committee (consisting of local government officials and nonprofit organizations) and to mentors assigned to the Bloustein School at Rutgers University from the Health Impact Project, a collaboration of the Robert Wood Johnson Foundation and The Pew Charitable Trusts, for review and comment, receiving some interesting suggestions. Then they prepared a final report, slides for briefings, and an executive summary.

Consistent with HIA practice, the team examined the impact of the process and study itself. The evaluation was by and large quite positive. The group noted one process limitation in that they had less access to ethnic minorities than they had hoped for. With time, they expect decision-makers to select some of their recommendations. They will use the proposed indicators to monitor disease, crime, and social and behavioral indicators to document the success of the project, although the effort will be difficult because of migration and other confounding factors.

Bloomfield Avenue Road Diet Evaluation

Located about 25 miles (about a 35-minute car drive) north of the Middlesex Greenway are the New Jersey towns of Bloomfield, Verona, Montclair, and Glen Ridge. They sit 16 miles west of the Empire State Building (about 50 minutes by car, much less on transit). These towns epitomize the variation possible in a small, largely suburban state with 565 municipal governments and about 8 million people. Each of these adjacent suburbs has a distinct ethnic/racial, age, and income mix. Glen Ridge and Verona are about 90 percent white, whereas Montclair and Bloomfield are about 60 percent white. Montclair has more black Americans than the other communities and Bloomfield has more Hispanics. The median income of Glen Ridge's residents is more than $150,000 annually; Montclair's and Verona's are about $100,000; and Bloomfield's is about $70,000.[28] Housing types, educational achievement, and other demographic indicators show that there are major distinctions among these four lower- to upper-middle-class towns. What they share is that all four are densely populated (106,000 people in their total 16.7 square miles or a density of 6,400 people per square mile).

The towns also share Bloomfield Avenue (County Road 506). This road runs from the southwest for 4.3 miles, crossing each of the four town centers and ending in Newark, the most populated city in New Jersey. Bloomfield Avenue is an undivided, four-lane highway marked by stop-and-go traffic as well as parallel parking along its edges. For those traveling on bicycles, as well as those trying to cross the avenue on foot, the experience is not pleasant and in places is downright treacherous.

New Jersey as a whole has a serious traffic safety problem, especially for pedestrians. Data support our perceptions. In 2008, according to the National Highway Traffic Safety

Administration's data, New Jersey ranked second in pedestrian deaths, behind only New York. In 2013, New Jersey's rank moved to third in the United States in pedestrian deaths behind New York and Nevada.[29,30]

In 2015, our group of university-based researchers, along with the four cities' government officials and not-for-profit groups, developed an HIA for the Bloomfield Avenue corridor. The goals were to identify, recommend, and evaluate changes in the roadway that would not only improve traffic flow but would also benefit nearby residents, walkers, bikers, and store owners.[28] The HIA focused on a "road diet" plan that would reduce the existing four lanes to three while adding turning lanes, protected bicycle lanes, and other safety-oriented changes. Six issues addressing the health effects were assessed:

1. Collisions with pedestrians, bicyclists, and drivers
2. Outdoor exposures to air pollution for pedestrians, bicyclists, and drivers
3. Mental health impacts associated with street and noise changes for pedestrians, bicyclists, and drivers
4. Social cohesion for communities along streets
5. Economic impacts along and near streets
6. Access to service, transit, and healthy food along the roadway

The road diet reconfiguration has the potential to decrease highway risk and, if it works as expected, should positively impact all of the attributes reviewed.

Methods

A steering committee consisting of 18 members representing 14 organizations from the four local governments, the county, business, health organizations, and bike/walk groups attended five meetings and worked with their members to provide input. The authors report that they used "Dotmocracy" (using dot stickers) in one of their sessions to locate traffic hot spots and high-risk places for walkers and bicyclists. The researchers took advantage of events to meet people, for example, at the Fine Arts and Crafts at Verona Park and the Montclair Bike Scavenger Hunt. An open house event was another opportunity to talk and listen. The group invited experts and officials to a roundtable session to discuss some of the scientific and engineering issues, such as obesity, physical activity, safety, and stress, They also interviewed local health department staff, and representatives of not-for-profit health organizations.

The research team reviewed the black and gray literature, obtaining data from the following sources:

- U.S. Census Bureau (population attributes)
- Behavioral Risk Factor Surveillance System for New Jersey

- County health departments
- Local police reports
- Traffic incident reports
- Local hospital and medical personnel
- NJ Department of Environmental Protection
- Local professionals who had local data from recent studies

The research team wrote a convenience survey and gathered survey data on paper and online. The survey had more than 80 questions focusing on people's uses of the roads and surrounding area, their perceptions, and concerns. People were recruited at public meetings, through email solicitation, and from postings on organization Web sites. More than 1,000 completed surveys were returned.

At the HIA screening stage, the research team used a checklist very similar to the one used in the greenway project focusing on the value of an HIA as a decision-aid tool, the feasibility of conducting the HIA within a six- to seven-month time frame, and receptiveness of the decision-makers to an HIA. An important point in this study was that Essex County manages this county road and, along with officials from the four towns, were open to acting on any recommendations generated by the process. Furthermore, community members welcomed this project as the first step in what they hoped would be a much larger study of each major road crossing. Overall, an HIA was conducted over about a six- to seven-month period, which permitted mapping and some new data, including gathering a convenience sample, interviewing, and discussion.

Results

The researchers drew half-mile radii around the highway and examined the four towns as a whole. They found 21 schools and determined that many students must cross Bloomfield Avenue to attend them. Three train stations and many bus stops are within one mile of the corridor. Nine senior living facilities are located along the avenue, as are three senior community centers and two farmer's markets. A road diet project should lead to reductions in auto accidents involving drivers, bikers, and pedestrians. Recommendations should lead to much a greater willingness of pedestrians to cross the road, and possibly to less air pollution.

Figure 5.2 is the causal pathway diagram linking the proposed road diet changes to safety improvements. The diagram focuses on benefits to pedestrians and bicycle riders, as well as those who would (1) increase their recreation, (2) gain access to a wider variety of food sources, and (3) gain physical access to health care services. These expectations can, in turn, be linked to 18 specific health outcomes such as hypertension, heart disease, and mental health.

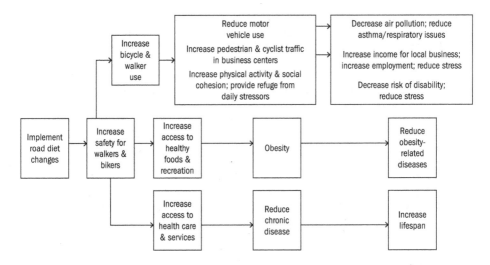

Source: Adapted from Lowrie et al. (2015).[28(p37)]

Figure 5.2. Causal Pathway Model of Road Diet on Safety Along Bloomfield Avenue

Another way of interpreting the expected benefits of the Bloomfield Avenue HIA is found in Table 5.5. The table summarizes the research team's findings about human health based in six specific areas for the target groups: pedestrians, bicyclists, drivers, seniors, the poor, storeowners, and the town residents as a whole. For instance, safety and stress reduction are expected to be the largest health benefits. Air pollution and access to transit and other services, as well as the local economy, were expected to be the least impacted.

As expected from a convenience sample, middle-aged and senior respondents who were extremely well educated were overrepresented in the results. With that caveat noted, a great deal of direction was provided by the surveys. Half of those respondents walk on Bloomfield Avenue and indicated they would walk more if they felt safer, and bicyclists said on average that they would make three or more additional bicycle trips along Bloomfield Avenue each month if it were safer. Disproportionately, those who said that they would walk were more likely to self-identify as Hispanic (64 percent) and black (69 percent) compared with white (49 percent). To walk more, they wanted better enforcement of traffic laws (67 percent), better pedestrian crossing signals (66 percent), and more time for pedestrians to cross the road with signals (52 percent). In regard to drivers, 39 percent said that when driving along Bloomfield Avenue they "often" feel more stress; another 51 percent said that they "sometimes" feel more stress.[28] In other words, 90 percent of respondents who drive on this stretch of road were stressed.

The combination of the data analysis, surveys, and public meetings provided some excellent insights upon which to base recommendations for the Bloomfield Avenue Road Diet. Specifically, 858 vehicle crashes were reported along the route (about 200 per mile) between 2009 and 2012. Pedestrians were involved in 46 of these. The HIA report

Table 5.5. Summary of Findings From Bloomfield Avenue Road Diet Evaluation

Health Outcome	Direction	Likelihood	Impact	Impacted Population
Safety	+	Likely	High	Drivers, pedestrians, and bicyclists
Physical activity	+	Possible	Medium	Town residents, especially lower-income and seniors
Air pollution	+	Possible	Low	Those who live or work within one block of the avenue, especially children and seniors
Stress	+	Likely	High	Drivers and commuters, shoppers, business patrons, and pedestrians
Social cohesion	+	Possible	Medium	Town residents
Local economy (more jobs and revenue)	+	Uncertain	Low	Business and property owners along the corridor and towns as a whole
Access to transit, service and food	+	Uncertain	Low	Residents of surrounding municipalities

Source: Adapted from Lowrie et al. (2015).[28(p60)]
Note: + = changes may improve health.

contains color maps of these events that show clear clusters or traffic safety hot spots that need to be addressed. Half of the survey respondents said that the route was not safe. Respondents identified cars stopped behind drivers waiting to parallel park (24%) and cars that were exiting from parking spaces (20%) as the most serious problems, followed by speeding (20%) and heavy traffic (18%). In regard to bicycling, more than 1 of 10 bicyclists said it was unsafe to cross and ride along Bloomfield Avenue. We provide three quotes from Lowrie et al. (2015):

1. Seniors from the Cooperative have trouble crossing Bloomfield and High Ave—a senior citizen was actually struck.
2. You have 6 seconds to cross the crosswalk, which is not long enough.
3. An 11 year old may be able to safely walk down Bloomfield Avenue, but may not have the skills to "navigate the madness." Kids don't pay attention to the crosswalk. Crossing guards definitely help.[28(p70)]

Recommendations

The HIA report offered 55 recommendations for improvements along the Bloomfield Avenue corridor. Those expected to have the highest positive impact are reproduced in Table 5.6. Having visited the area on multiple occasions, we can testify to the need for these measures, especially those related to traffic calming and crosswalk safety.

Table 5.6. Selected Recommendations From the Bloomfield Avenue Road Diet Evaluation

Institute Measures to Slow Motor Vehicle Speeds and Reduce Unsafe Driving
• Institute traffic calming measures including lane reduction. • Consider more frequent police patrol for speed and traffic violations. • Add more speed limit signs or speed limit paint on the roadways at key locations. • Consider installing radar feedback speed limit signs.
Improve crosswalk safety
• Make crosswalks more prominent with high-visibility paint. • Reduce crossing length through lane reductions, curb extensions, and/or pedestrian refuge islands. • Carefully study crossing times and make improvements to ensure adequate length of time for all pedestrians to cross. • Install countdown signals at every signalized intersection, with pedestrian lead intervals. • Consider vibrotactile/audible signals to meet ADA standards. • Consider flashing signals or beacons at unsignalized or mid-block crossings. • Consider increasing the number of crossing guards at strategic times and locations, with a priority to assist children and senior citizens. • Continue to use "cops in the crosswalk" stings, and adopt new statewide crossing guard training methods. • Minimize turning conflicts with drivers and pedestrians with no right on red restrictions where possible.
Promote Driver, Pedestrian, and Bicycle Safety Education
• Promote local driver safety initiatives including Courteous Driving Pledge, Drive with Care Montclair, New Jersey Transportation Planning Authority's Street Smart Challenge, and Vision Zero. • Support local efforts to educate pedestrians and cyclists about safety, prioritizing youth, seniors, and low-income populations. • Provide lights and safety vests to low-income/low-industry workers who use bicycles for travel to and from work.
Promote Alternatives to Driving
• Reconfigure travel lanes to add protected bicycle lanes and infrastructure. • Promote use of public transportation operation through increased awareness of schedules, routes, and fares. • Upgrade transit sites (prominence, condition of shelter or benches, etc.). • Identify ways to transport residents, especially seniors and people with disabilities, with additional shuttle, trolleys, jitneys, etc. • Educate residents on transit schedules and stop locations. Make senior shuttle routes and times more prominent. • Educate residents on features of transit (kneeling busses) and how to use the bike racks on buses.
Improve Feeling of Security
• Improve pedestrian scale lighting in strategic areas. • Increase police patrols in certain target areas where perceived or actual crime is higher. • Consider security cameras and post notices about them. • Conduct a Crime Prevention through Environmental Design analysis to identify ways to modify the built environment to improve safety from crime.

Source: Adapted from Lowrie et al. (2015).[28(p61)]

Consistent with HIA practice, the team reviewed the process and designed a monitoring plan. The final product includes suggestions on how the value of the HIA could be enhanced by collecting more field data—particularly on walking, bicycling, and vehicular traffic—to provide input on crosswalk and traffic improvement design priorities. The report also suggests collecting additional data about air pollution as it impacts seniors, the disabled, and other vulnerable populations.

Final Thoughts

We cannot think of a local public health issue that would not benefit from the application of the three types of tools presented in this chapter. There are, however, challenges to using them in a cookbook fashion. For example, legal and political considerations differ across locations and the differences may require the second-level questions in a checklist to be altered to fit those situations. Surveys and other methods of gathering or disseminating public information are, to some extent, the products of local expectations, what governments will permit, and what researchers are familiar with. Suffice it to say that methods that are widely used and considered standard in some places are not going to work in others.

The great strength of the HIA is the dedication to being transparent and involving stakeholders. Compared with an EIS or risk analysis (see Chapters 8 and 9), detail is somewhat sacrificed in an HIA. On the other hand, HIAs can provide timely results, particularly for health-related decisions that do not need such exacting detail. We expect that gradually HIAs will find their way into EISs as tools for decision-makers to gain a better understanding of public and community issues that are, in our opinion, not adequately represented in EISs and are absent in risk assessments.

References

1. Greenberg M, Belnay G, Cesanek W, Neuman N, Hepherd G. *A Primer on Industrial Environmental Impact.* New Brunswick, NJ: Center for Urban Policy Research, Rutgers University; 1979.

2. Greenberg MR, Weiner MD. Keeping surveys valid, reliable, and useful: a tutorial. *Risk Anal.* 2014;34(8):1362–1375.

3. Greenberg MR. *The Environmental Impact Statement After Two Generations: Managing Environmental Power.* New York, NY: Routledge; 2013.

4. Greenberg M, Burger J, Powers C, et al. Choosing remediation and waste management options at hazardous and radioactive waste sites. *Remediat J.* 2002;13(1):39–58.

5. Dillman DA, Smyth JD, Christian LM. *Internet, Mail, and Mixed-Mode Surveys: The Tailored Design Method*. 3rd ed. New York, NY: Wiley; 2008.

6. Fowler FJ. *Survey Research Methods (Applied Social Research Methods Series, No. 1)*. Thousand Oaks, CA: Sage; 2013.

7. Rea LM, Parker RA. *Designing and Conducting Survey Research: A Comprehensive Guide*. 3rd ed. San Francisco, CA: John Wiley & Sons; 2005.

8. Weiner M, Puniello O. Consider the non-adopter: developing a prediction model for the adoption of household-level broadband access. *Socioecon Plann Sci*. 2012;46:183–193.

9. Krueger R, Casey M. *Focus Groups: A Practical Guide for Applied Research*. Thousand Oaks, CA: Sage; 2015.

10. Morgan D. *Focus Groups as Qualitative Research*. 2nd ed. Qualitative Research Methods Series 16. Thousand Oaks, CA: Sage; 1997.

11. Chess C, Purcell K. Public participation and the environment: do we know what works? *Environ Sci Technol*. 1999;33(16):2685–2692.

12. McComas KA. Public meetings about local waste management problems: comparing participants to nonparticipants. *Environ Manage*. 2001;27(1):135–147.

13. McComas K. Citizen satisfaction with public meetings used for risk communication. *J Appl Commun Res*. 2003;31(2):164–184.

14. Greenberg M, Lowrie K. A proposed model for community participation and risk communication for a DOE-led stewardship program. *Fed Facil Environ J*. 2001;Spring:125–141.

15. Eccleston CH. *Environmental Impact Assessment: A Guide to Best Professional Practices*. Boca Raton, FL: CRC Press; 2011.

16. Turnbull RH, ed. *Environmental and Health Impact Assessment of Development Projects: A Handbook for Practitioners*. Abingdon, England: Taylor and Francis; 1992.

17. Ross D, Orenstein M, Botchwey N. *Health Impact Assessment in the United States*. New York, NY: Springer; 2014.

18. Kemm J. *Health Impact Assessment: Past Achievement, Current Understanding, and Future Progress*. New York, NY: Oxford University Press; 2013.

19. Birley M. *Health Impact Assessment: Principles and Practice*. London, England: Earthscan; 2011.

20. International Council on Mining and Metals. Good practice guidance on health impact assessment. 2010. Available at: https://www.icmm.com/website/publications/pdfs/977.pdf. Accessed June 19, 2017.

21. The Society of Practitioners of Health Impact. SOPHIA Assessment. 2014. Available at: http://hiasociety.org. Accessed April 26, 2016.

22. International Association for Impact Assessment. Health impact assessment blog. Available at: http://healthimpactassessment.blogspot.com. Accessed April 26, 2016.

23. International Association for Impact Assessment. The leading global network on impact assessment. 2016. Available at: http://www.iaia.org. Accessed April 26, 2016.

24. National Association of County and City Health Officials. Planning for healthy places with health impact assessments. Available at: http://archived.naccho.org/topics/environmental/health-impact-assessment. Accessed March 7, 2017.

25. IMPACT. International Health Impact Assessment Consortium. Available at: https://www.liverpool.ac.uk/psychology-health-and-society/research/impact/about. Accessed May 1, 2016.

26. High-speed railroading. *The Economist.* July 22, 2010. Available at: http://www.economist.com/node/16636101. Accessed April 26, 2016.

27. Lowrie K, Von Hagen L, Sewell E. Middlesex County Access Plan: health impact assessment. Planning Healthy Communities Initiative. 2014. Available at: http://njhic.rutgers.edu/middlesex-county-access-plan-health-impact-assessment. Accessed April 26, 2016.

28. Lowrie K, Von Hagen L, Sewell E. Bloomfield Ave. complete corridor health impact assessment. Planning Healthy Communities Initiative. 2015. Available at: http://phci.rutgers.edu/bloomfield-avenue-hia. Accessed April 26, 2016.

29. National Highway Traffic Safety Administration. NHTSA traffic safety facts 2013 data. 2015. Available at: http://www-nrd.nhtsa.dot.gov/Pubs/812196.pdf. Accessed April 26, 2016.

30. National Highway Traffic Safety Administration. NHTSA traffic safety facts 2008 data. Available at: http://www-nrd.nhtsa.dot.gov/Pubs/812196.pdf. Accessed April 26, 2016.

6

KEEPING PEOPLE OUT OF HARM'S WAY

The context for this chapter is all too common. Imagine that you just had a call from the mayor's office. A local developer has proposed an assisted living facility for senior citizens and disabled persons in your town. The site is a lovely wooded area about 300 feet back from a small coastal beach. It seems perfect, with beautiful views for the residents, birds chirping early in the morning, and occasional strolls along a planned boardwalk. There is also fishing, swimming, and wading, and just sitting under an umbrella enjoying the weather and the scenery. In short, the developer says that it is a great place for people who can afford to pay for a beautiful location and the needed assistance. Furthermore, there are no neighbors. Thus, no one has objected—so far.

You recall that the proposed site has been struck by tropical storms, although not within the past decade. You also understand that keeping people out of harm's way includes thinking about and preventing the consequences of rare events that can kill and injure people and destroy assets. Does it make sense to locate an assisted living facility in this place? You might think the location would better serve the community as open space. However, the reality is that developers with a great deal of money and political access can usually find a way to get what they want. The developer will strongly argue that the site can be protected against storms and you may be required to approve a site plan with facilities that can withstand all but the worst possible storm. You must accept an overall design that will allow the site to return to normal or to a new normal as soon as possible after a severe storm. The overall design may include a new sea wall, which will help the developer but might not be sufficient to stop high waves and will likely cause increased flooding in adjacent areas.

To provide responsible parties with constructive, science-informed suggestions, analysts need to answer the following three risk analysis questions (see Chapter 8 for additional discussion on risk analysis):

1. What are the most consequential risks?
2. Who is at risk, where, and when from these consequential risks?
3. What can be done to prevent exposure and to help people return to normal or close to normal if the event occurs?

This chapter presents and illustrates three tools that should be part of your effort to keep people out of harm's way:

1. Accessing and interpreting population data.
2. Mapping as a way of communicating information.
3. Conducting a hazard mitigation analysis.

These tools are illustrated by case studies that examine efforts underway in the State of Texas. Within Texas, the Houston–Galveston area is considered the most vulnerable of all the state's regions, especially Galveston City, which is located on a barrier island in the Gulf of Mexico.

Accessing and Interpreting Population Data

It is important to know where vulnerable people and assets are located. The U.S. Census Bureau publishes population data at the national, state, county, and local government levels, with estimates of persons in neighborhoods, by using census tract and block data. The authors have used census data since the late 1960s, and we can unequivocally state that the population data readily available today are nothing short of amazing compared with a half-century ago. We can quickly access data about the nation, states, cities, and other local governments, census tracts, blocks, zip code areas, and special areas such as congressional districts.

In the late 1960s, when the first author wrote his master's thesis, his analysis involved using census tract data (areas of about 5,000 people that the U.S. Census Bureau drew a boundary around to approximate neighborhoods). Data were available only in large paper volumes. Data consisting of about 300 census tracts had to be key-punched on IBM cards, which were then fed into the "mainframe" computer at Columbia University. Preparing the data took weeks; analyzing it, less time. Fifty years later, we can access data on our desktop screen and the raw data can be downloaded to a spreadsheet in a matter of 5 to 10 minutes. Not only are current data available, but intercensus estimates also can be accessed, and the U.S. Census Bureau provides software to map some of the data. We are not saying that there is no work involved to access the data. However, if you work through the U.S. Census Bureau's various files or if you know someone that is already familiar with accessing files, you can obtain data sets that will allow you to assess the geography of vulnerable people.

Specifically, we suggest the following data fields to identify relatively vulnerable people:

- Over 65 years old, especially over 75 years
- Less than 5 years old
- Without an automobile

- Disabled, pre-existing health conditions and other conditions requiring special care
- Not able to communicate in English
- Poor (assuming limited assets if a hazardous event occurs)
- Lack of knowledge of the area (measured by rapid population change, rental status, summer visitor)

An area with high concentrations of these individuals ranks high in relative vulnerability. Although not all of these data can be obtained from the census, much of it can. The U.S. Census Bureau also samples some of the U.S. population every year, providing inter-censal estimates. If you type "factfinder" into a search engine, it will send you to the U.S. Census Bureau Web site, which can provide you access to a great deal of the most recent data for states, counties, metropolitan areas, and larger cities.

In a series of papers and reports, Susan Cutter[1] and colleagues established a logic of how to identify socially vulnerable populations. Using county data, the team included the data fields in the bulleted list above, as well as others, and employed a statistical tool called factor analysis to cluster the results (an example will follow). The South Carolina group then ranked the counties in the United States with regard to social vulnerability.[2]

Although Cutter's important work showed that the county level is a good scale at which to start, neighborhood (census tract) and block-scale data are a must to identify how to keep people out of harm's way. For example, we need to know precisely how many people live in the 100-year flood plain, near areas vulnerable to high winds, and in places that have suffered mud slides or other hazard events.

To identify clusters of high-risk people at the neighborhood and block scales, you need to obtain the raw data from the census files, which will require some hard work. For example, it took us only 10 minutes to obtain census data for the State of Michigan, the county that hosts Detroit and Detroit itself. Yet it took the authors more than three hours to download the raw census data for these places so that it could be analyzed with factor analysis and cluster analysis (another statistical method that is typically used to analyze spatial data) at the census tract scale.

A relatively simple illustration should help. The authors have long been interested in the relationship between segregation by socioeconomic status, race, ethnicity, and health and urban service delivery (e.g., shopping, transportation, access to health providers) and vulnerability.[3] For example, we wanted to determine if borders between big cities and their suburban neighbors were socially permeable—that is, one side of the border did not have a distinct population and the other side, in a different municipality, a markedly different one. Using the census data from 1970, 1980, 1990, and 2000, we compared attributes of the census tracts within one mile of the borders of Chicago, Illinois; Detroit, Michigan; Los Angeles, California; New York, New York; and Philadelphia, Pennsylvania, with their immediate suburbs. Census data were obtained about educational achievement, income, housing value, rents, and type of employment, unemployment rates, and other indicators. In all of the cities, the borders were typically marked by cemeteries,

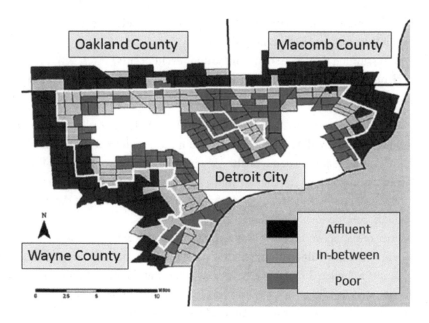

Source: Based on data from Greenberg 2009.[3]
Figure 6.1. Detroit Border Residential Segregation Study

shopping malls, parks, golf courses, rivers, and highways. None of the borders were permeable, as illustrated by Detroit in Figure 6.1. The map shows only census tracts within a mile of the city–suburban border—the white line. Note that the Detroit border provides a striking socioeconomic barrier between the city and its suburbs.

We could not have done this analysis without the raw census data, which required an investment in both time and expertise. Was the investment worth the benefit? For us the answer is yes because once the data are downloaded, they can be easily updated and used for various projects. For the uninitiated, the initial foray into using raw census data can be tedious and time consuming. We recommend getting help from someone with experience. It should only take about an hour to learn the basics of accessing census files.

Another example of the use of census data to define populations at risk comes from Pflicke and colleagues.[4] The team used census tract data to identify populations vulnerable to storms and floods in New Jersey. They used factor analysis to identify clusters of vulnerable people by using the vulnerability metrics listed earlier in this chapter. Those clusters were then overlain on maps of likely flood zones and wave height zones. The resulting maps allowed officials to find the populations most vulnerable to tropical storms among the state's 8 million people living in 2,100 census tracts.

A final point must be made about defining populations at risk. The previously mentioned examples focus on where people live, not where they work or travel through. From a risk analyst's perspective, everyone touched by a location is potentially exposed to risk, regardless of the time spent at the locale. For instance, residents may be at risk 20 to 24 hours a day, seven days a week. Workers may be at risk 8 hours a day, five days a week. Do not fail to consider the driver who passes through the risk area for 30 seconds each day, five times a week. These populations are all at risk.

We urge you to consider every possible case of exposure to avoid missing a vulnerable population. For example, the first author worked on siting new nuclear power plants during the period when that was still happening in the United States. He and his colleagues attempted to estimate the residential, worker, and traveler populations. The worker population contributed significantly to the at-risk population, even after weighting their presence in the area by time. This led to major debates about what the regulations really meant by the term "population at risk."

Mapping as a Way of Communicating Information

The availability of high-speed computers and user-friendly statistical and mapping packages means that you do not need a professional cartographer to make a map, which is good. Unfortunately, many maps produced are not good; they are confusing at best and inaccurate at worst because those producing them are not familiar with the basics of cartography. The following three reasons stand out as leading causes of misleading information displayed on maps:

1. Misuse of colors and symbols
2. Misuse of types of maps
3. Overlaying data that may or may not be causally related

If you want to get attention, use red, orange, and yellow. If you want to dampen concern, then use blue and green. An area with significantly higher risk than average probably should be red, orange, or yellow. But if the highest rates are only slightly higher than the average, then it is questionable whether you should use provocative colors. The opposite is also true—that is, just because an area has among the lowest risk rates does not mean that the population should not act to reduce its risk. Similarly, you should not use symbols such as a skull and crossbones, snakes, sharks, or other inappropriate signage on a map.

The type of map matters. For example, imagine a physically large rural county that has a single high-hazard area in the southeast corner. The analyst knows that the risk is limited to a small area around the site. But the risk is displayed in a choropleth map (one that uses differences in coloring or symbols within the entire census area to indicate risk). This kind of map will lead to major overstatement of the spatial extent of the risk.

One of the most painful mistakes to avoid is overlaying data sets on maps that lead the public to believe that two attributes are causally related. For example, the first author was involved in a distressing incident when someone with outstanding medical credentials but limited geographical ones produced a map showing that city cancer death rates over-lapped closely on a map of landfills. The assumption drawn by some viewers was that the landfills caused these cancers. And although that possibility cannot be entirely dismissed, no one in the area drank water that came from this area, no one had physical contact with the landfills, and, hence, an actual physical link between outcome and inferred cause was misleading. In other words, two or more attributes that appear to co-exist in place do not necessarily share a causal relationship. It is important not to give that impression when communicating risk.[5,6]

By contrast, a map that shows the location of people who would need to be evacuated if a tropical storm hit an area can legitimately be overlain on a map of storm surge prob-abilities. That is, the storm surge could require evacuation of the population at risk in that area. This is clearly a relationship that should be shown on a map.

With these caveats noted, our capability to make two- and three-dimensional maps is already remarkable and increasing. It is common for public health and planning students to take at least one course and preferably two mapping and related data and communica-tions courses. Overall, census demographic, health, and land use data statistical analysis and mapping are increasingly being combined to inform hazard mitigation planning.

Hazard Mitigation Analysis

The Stafford Act of 1988 created a system whereby a presidential disaster declaration or an emergency declaration triggered physical and financial assistance through the Federal Emergency Management Agency (FEMA). Although that act required hazard mitigation plans, the plans were not systematically evaluated and funds provided were not linked to the plans.[7] By 2000, it had become clear that economic losses from natural hazard events across the nation were markedly increasing and Congress passed the Disaster Mitigation Act (DMA).[8] The short-term goal of the DMA was to more efficiently respond to major disasters. The long-term objective was to reduce loss of life and property by proactively encouraging hazard mitigation planning at the state and local levels. It was simply increasingly costly to continue to react to events that had already occurred.

The DMA and accompanying regulations and policies have changed how government and private concerns think about hazards and vulnerability. States must assist local gov-ernments with building partnerships that lead to integrated planning so that local gov-ernments have coordinated and effective risk management options. Procedurally, state and local governments write the plans for hazard mitigation, and these must be approved by FEMA. Then, using priorities set forth in the approved plan, federal and other funds are applied to reduce vulnerability and improve resilience.[9–16]

While individual counties, groups of counties, cities, and townships assume the major local responsibility for risk management, in our experience it is the state governments that play a key role in setting the agenda, describing expectations, and then working hard to build cooperation. With some exceptions, a local government is going to be hard pressed to make effective hazard mitigation plans without good guidance from state government.

FEMA wants hazard mitigation plans and planning to end the cycle of disaster damage, reconstruction, and repeated damage. Indeed, the agency spells out what it expects hazard mitigation plans to do for state, tribal, and local governments:

- Increase education and awareness around threats, hazards, and vulnerabilities.
- Build partnerships for risk reduction involving government, organizations, businesses, and the public.
- Identify long-term, broadly supported strategies for risk reduction.
- Align risk reduction with other state, tribal, or community objectives.
- Identify implementation approaches that focus resources on the greatest risks and vulnerabilities.
- Communicate priorities to potential sources of funding.[15]

Can planning accomplish these ambitious goals? That is a legitimate question as the United States has a strong tradition of home-rule. Despite the challenge, the evaluation of plans has expanded since the mid-1990s, leading many local officials to conclude that good plans lead to better results, including hazard mitigation plans.[17-22] Effective plans have the following six elements:

1. Goals reflecting local values
2. Risk assessments and risk management options grounded in sound science
3. Policies written to guide decisions and implementation
4. Organizational and financial support throughout the process
5. Interorganizational throughout
6. Meaningful participation from the beginning

The legal basis for FEMA's proactive mitigation planning program is found in federal laws, regulations, and policies. At the heart of these is that FEMA requires state, tribal, and local governments to prepare and adopt hazard mitigation plans as a precondition for receiving many types of nonemergency disaster assistance, including money for hazard mitigation projects. Secondly, jurisdictions must update their hazard mitigation plans and resubmit them for FEMA review and approval every five years to maintain eligibility for federal government support. Finally, FEMA provides planning grants to support state, tribal, and local government efforts to develop and update their mitigation plans.

Space does not permit a full discussion of the laws, regulations, policies, and programs related to hazard mitigation planning. Instead, Table 6.1 lists some of the key ones. These will lead you to others, and we also suggest reviewing the U.S. Environmental Protection Agency's Web site, which includes information about its sustainability programs, global

Table 6.1. Selected Laws, Regulations, Policies, and Programs Governing Hazard Mitigation Planning

Law, Regulation, Policy, or Program	Comments
Robert T. Stafford Disaster Relief and Emergency Assistance Act as amended by the Disaster Mitigation Act of 2000	This act provides the legal authority for states, local governments, and tribal nations to undertake risk assessments and risk management programs.
Hazard Mitigation Grant Program	Under the Stafford Act, resources are provided to communities to implement hazard mitigation measures after a presidential major disaster declaration; program also funds hazard mitigation plan updates.
Pre-disaster Mitigation Grant Program	Under the Stafford Act, program provides planning and project grants to update hazard mitigation plans and build hazard mitigation programs.
Public Assistance Grant Program	Under the Stafford Act, program provides funds to help governments and certain nonprofit organizations to respond to and recover from major disasters.
Fire Management Assistance Grant Program	This program provides assistance to governments in order to mitigate fires on public and private forests and grasslands that threaten to become disasters.
National Flood Insurance Act of 1968	This act provides funding to governments for planning and development of hazard mitigation plans and projects.
Sandy Recovery Improvement Act of 2013	This act amends the Stafford Act to allow recognized tribal governments the option to request a presidential emergency or major disaster declaration independent of a state government.
Title 44, Chapter 1, Part 201 of the Code of Federal Regulations	This section provides regulations, requirements, and procedures to implement the hazard mitigation planning provisions of the Stafford Act.
State Mitigation Plan Review Guide	FEMA document 101659 explains FEMA's expectations for state plans.
Local Mitigation Plan Review Guide	FEMA document 23194 explains FEMA's expectations for local plans.
Tribal Multihazard Mitigation Planning Guidance	FEMA document 29677 explains FEMA's expectations for tribal nations.

Source: Based on data from Federal Emergency Management Agency.[15]
Note: FEMA = Federal Emergency Management Agency.

climate change efforts, environmental justice programs, and joint efforts with FEMA (see Chapter 11).

Readers of this book may have neither the inclination nor the time to review all the laws, regulations, policies, and programs. Thus, Table 6.2 contains a short list of FEMA document library resources that we recommend. Simply type FEMA into a search engine and, once on the Web site, search for the resource.

Despite the external appearance of great complexity, multiple laws, regulations, policies, programs, and documents, in reality the hazard mitigation planning process can be divided into five steps for local governments:

1. Organize information about internal and external assets available for mitigation.
2. Assess vulnerabilities and risks.

3. Develop a mitigation plan.
4. Implement plan and monitor progress.
5. Repeat the first four steps to update and modify the plan.

As of 2016, all 50 states, the District of Columbia, Guam, American Samoa, Northern Marianna Islands, Puerto Rico, and the U.S. Virgin Islands had FEMA-approved state mitigation plans. Notably, 22,601 local governments had FEMA-approved or approvable-pending-adoption local mitigation plans and 140 tribal governments had current tribal mitigation plans. These plans cover more than 80 percent of the U.S. population.[15] The process of cooperative planning between states and groups of local governments clearly is underway.

In summary, the federal government created a financially and politically acceptable framework to allow state and local governments and selective private organizations

Table 6.2. Federal Emergency Management Agency Document Resources for Practitioners

Resource	FEMA Document Number and Comment
Local Mitigation Planning Handbook	Document 31598 offers quite a few suggestions and examples the communities can use together or to update their hazard mitigation plans.
State Mitigation Planning Key Topics Bulletins	Document 115780 provides short documents providing ideas and resources for state officials to use for updating state plans.
State Mitigation Plan Review Guide Fact Sheet	Document 101659 provides a summary of FEMA's hazard mitigation planning program.
Tribal Planning Fact Sheet	Document 18375 is the fact sheet for tribal governments.
Plan Integration: Linking Local Planning Efforts	Document 108893 is a carefully written, step-by-step guide to help communities develop and modify their plans.
Integrating Hazard Mitigation into Local Planning: Case Studies and Tools for Community Officials (see also accompanying fact sheets)	Document 31372 is intended to help local officials incorporate risk mitigation into their existing plans, codes, and programs.
Planning for a Sustainable Future	Document 2110 speaks to integrating sustainability ideas into hazard mitigation processes.
Rebuilding for a More Sustainable Future: An Operational Framework	Document 767 is a broader look into the need to integrate human health, economy, the environment, and social well-being into hazard mitigation planning.
Hazard Mitigation: Integrating Best Practices and Planning	Document 19261, written by the American Planning Association, speaks to the need of local planning officials to integrate standard planning with hazard mitigation planning.
Planning for Post-Disaster Recovery and Reconstruction	Document 2147 is a widely used report prepared by the American Planning Association with many examples about how standard planning can interface with hazard mitigation planning.

Note: FEMA = Federal Emergency Management Agency. To access these reports, type "FEMA reports" into a search engine and then enter the number.

to reduce the likelihood of people being killed or injured and of assets being destroyed from a disaster event.

A Tiered Case Study: The State of Texas, Houston–Galveston Area, and Galveston City

Unfortunately, people have not been kept out of harm's way in many places across the United States. Several reports have ranked the riskiest of these places. For example, Whiteman[23] offered the following list of the 10 riskiest states, including the number of major disaster declarations each has experienced since 1953:

1. Texas (88)
2. California (79)
3. Oklahoma (75)
4. New York (68)
5. Florida (67)
6. Louisiana (60)
7. Alabama (58)
8. Arkansas (58)
9. Kentucky (56)
10. Missouri (55)

All of these states are geographically large, seven are coastal states, and the other three have been struck by multiple floods and tornadoes. Note the 88 major disaster declarations in Texas since 1953. One or more disasters has been declared in Texas nearly every year since 1953—tornadoes, floods, wildfires, coastal storms, and even a fertilizer plant explosion.

In 2012, Climate Central identified the five U.S. cities and metropolitan regions most vulnerable to hurricanes[24]:

1. Tampa–St. Petersburg, Florida
2. Miami, Florida
3. New Orleans, Louisiana
4. Norfolk–Virginia Beach, Virginia
5. Houston–Galveston, Texas

Although published before Superstorm Sandy devastated parts of New Jersey and New York City, Climate Central observed that "pretty much any location along the Gulf and East Coasts are fair game for hurricanes to strike." Climate Central also noted that the Galveston–Houston area has 6.1 million people, along with vital oil and gas infrastructure sitting on low-lying land that has been subject to tropical storms every 9 to 16 years. Hurricane Ike hit the area in 2008, causing 20 deaths and $27.8 billion in damage.

Pickles[25] identified the 10 U.S. cities and metropolitan areas most likely to suffer natural disasters. Note that 9 of the 10 are in the South, which is highly vulnerable to hurricanes, flooding, earthquakes, tornadoes, and wildfires.

1. Fayetteville, North Carolina
2. Rome, Georgia
3. Birmingham, Alabama
4. Anniston, Alabama
5. Riverside–San Bernardino–Ontario, California
6. Columbia, South Carolina
7. Augusta–Richmond, South Carolina–Georgia border
8. Tuscaloosa, Alabama
9. Hattiesburg, Mississippi
10. Jackson, Mississippi

The most populous of the contiguous U.S. states are Texas, California, and Florida—states that have been grappling with natural hazards for decades. Each has considerable industrial activity that is placed at risk during a storm and that can also be a source of risk itself. To illustrate the use of the tools and demonstrate the daunting challenge of keeping people out of harm's way, we have chosen Texas and present a three-tiered case study at the state, metropolitan region, and city levels.

Tier 1: Texas, a Multihazard Challenge

Texas is a massive state of 267,000 square miles (691,000 square kilometers). Only sparsely populated Alaska is larger. Texas has 12 river basins, some of which are large (e.g., Rio Grande and Brazos) and others small (e.g., Cypress, Lavaca). The rivers themselves do not necessarily lead to a higher probability of flooding. Rather, it is the state's terrain and climate that are the major predictive factors for natural disasters.[26]

The southeast Gulf Coast of Texas averages 55 inches of precipitation per year, whereas 796 miles (1281 kilometers) to the west in El Paso (about an 11-hour drive; we recommend flying) it is only about 9 inches. The state's Gulf Coast shore line is 367 miles long with 17 barrier beaches, some of which are heavily used. Overall, Texas's climate, terrain, geology, soils, and other physical attributes are remarkably variable and pose a severe challenge for state and local hazard mitigation planners.[26]

Added to its physical diversity, Texas has a large population that has been growing more rapidly than that of other states. Specifically, between the years 2000 and 2015, the Texas population grew almost 32 percent. Only Nevada, Utah, and Arizona grew relatively more. Texas's population was about 27.5 million in 2015, an absolute increase of 7 million since 2000, more than any other state. Furthermore, much of the population increase is being added in the highly vulnerable triangle formed by Dallas–Fort Worth (Tarrant County) in the north, Houston–Galveston (Harris County) in the southeast, and San Antonio (Bexar County) in the southwest.[27]

Given the complex physical, legal, and social environment of Texas, the state must play a critical role as intermediary between FEMA's programs and requirements and local government priorities. Berke et al.[28] studied the hazard mitigation plans of all states and rated each according to six categories:

1. Goals
2. Fact base
3. Mitigation policy
4. Implementation and monitoring
5. Interagency coordination
6. Participation

Texas ranked among the top states in goals and participation. As the state with the most presidential disaster declarations between 1953 and 2011, the 2013 Texas plan listed the following 15 priority natural hazards in rank order:

1. Floods
2. Hurricanes
3. Wildfire
4. Tornado
5. Drought
6. Coastal erosion
7. Dam/levee failure
8. Earthquakes
9. Expansive soil
10. Extreme heat
11. Hailstorm
12. Land subsidence
13. Severe winter storms
14. Windstorms
15. Lightning[25]

Figure 6.2 is a geographical portrait of the five highest priority hazards noted in the 2010–2013 Texas Hazard Mitigation Plan.[26] Note that the triangle linking the Dallas–Fort Worth, Houston, and San Antonio areas is vulnerable to all five major hazards, and some counties within that area are vulnerable to two or three and some of the others on the main Texas hazards list.

Floods, the highest ranked hazard in Texas, number about 400 per year. Floods are a chronic and sometimes acute problem in Texas, mostly along the coast and in central

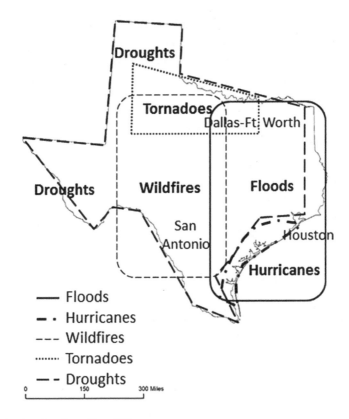

Source: Based on data from State of Texas.[26,29]
Figure 6.2. The Geography of Texas's Five Major Hazard Concerns

part of the state. The Hazard Mitigation Report notes that more than 90 percent of damage costs attributable to disasters in Texas are flood-related. Furthermore, no part of the state escapes the problems and consequences of flooding.

Storm surges and fierce winds from hurricanes and tropical storms are the second-ranked hazard for Texas. These can cause enormous numbers of deaths and injuries. The Gulf Coast is clearly the most vulnerable, but 22 counties (including some not directly on the coast) have been severely damaged.

Wildfires account for the number-three ranking of hazards in Texas. The wildfire area is directly west of the flood zone and, in fact, some counties are in both zones. The mitigation plan suggests that damage associated with wildfires is understated because there are no standards for reporting, and, accordingly, many wildfires go unreported to authorities.

As we move down the hazard rank list, Texas is hit by about 125 tornadoes each year, primarily in the north-central part of the state in the Red River Valley and north of the Dallas–Fort Worth area (hazard rank number four). Not to be ignored, as Figure 6.2 shows, nearly the entire state of Texas is at risk of drought (number five).

We have studied many state hazard mitigation plans and, along with California, Texas faces the widest variety of hazard-related challenges. The sheer size and variety of hazards requires a broad range of expertise and representation from across the state in order to set priorities. Thus, the following Texas agencies or authorities were heavily involved in building the state's hazard mitigation plan:

- Division of Emergency Management
- Texas A&M Forest Service
- Commission on Environmental Quality
- Department of Insurance
- Department of Transportation
- General Land Office
- Water Development Board
- Railroad Commission

Texas also added a technical assistance group with participants from Texas A&M, Texas Tech, the University of North Texas, the University of Texas, the Texas Geographic Society, and the Emergency Management Association of Texas.

Texas is among the strongest of the home-rule states. Toward that end, the Texas state group sent a questionnaire to local governments for input. We summarize key elements of those questions here:

- Hazards
    o What are your major natural and local hazards?
    o For each of these, what is the number of structures at risk?
    o What is the value of these structures?
    o What damage should be expected from a mid-range severe event?
- Change in hazards during past five years
    o Has there been a change in the population?
    o Has the inventory of structures changed?
    o Has there been a change in the severity of damage?
- Local capability
    o Are there building codes?
    o Is there zoning?
    o Are there land use controls?
    o Are there other policies that impact property vulnerability?
    o Is there compliance with the National Flood Insurance Program?
    o Is there compliance with fire protection and building codes?
    o Is there sufficient local budget, administrative and technical staff?
    o Is there a political focus on hazard mitigation?

The Texas report notes that, over time, more responsibility for data and decisions will come from the 254 counties in the form of county and local plans for hazard mitigation.

In addition, major regional groups will be reviewing all those plans. The overall goal of the review process is to identify areas with the highest priorities for mitigation in order to guide federal funding to those areas with high priorities and good mitigation plans.

Tier 2: Houston–Galveston Hazard Mitigation Planning

Hazard mitigation plans focus on natural hazards; however, technological hazard events may also impact a state or region. Table 6.3 shows that hypothetical worst events for Texas as listed in the state's 2013 Hazard Mitigation Report Update.[29] Note that six of the eight events would be natural hazard events and two would be technological. Geographically, six of the eight events are in the Dallas–Fort Worth–Houston–San Antonio triangle (see Figure 6.2) and three are in the Houston–Galveston area.

Another way of showing the concentration of vulnerability and risk in Texas is to examine repetitive insurance losses over time. In its year 2013 Hazard Mitigation Report Update,[29] Texas listed more than 20,000 repetitive loss cases throughout the state. These losses were located in 143 of the state's 254 counties, and they were not randomly distributed. Fifty-five percent of the insurance losses were in Harris County (including Houston) and another 12 percent were in Galveston County. In other words, these two adjacent counties accounted for two-thirds of the repetitive loss payments in Texas through February 2013. For comparative purposes, these counties accounted for only 17 percent of the state's population. Another way of saying this is that these two counties had four times as many repetitive damage-related insurance claims as people.

Delving deeper into the repetitive loss data, Harris County has 14 times as many people as Galveston County, but only 4.4 times as many repetitive loss payments.

Table 6.3. Hypothetical Worst-Case Hazard Events for Texas

Type of Hazard	Hypothetical Event	Location and Time
Natural	Category 5 hurricane	Galveston Island, Labor Day weekend
	Rain and category 4 hurricane and tornado	Rio Grande Valley on July 4
	Multiple tornadoes	Dallas–Ft. Worth, spring weekend
	Extreme drought, and high winds and wildfires	San Angelo, Travis counties in August
	Heavy rainfall leading to flash flooding	El Paso, summer months
	Influenza virus pandemic	Houston, February
Technological	Structural dam failure and interruption of transportation or utility systems	Dallas–Ft. Worth—no time specified
	Railroad chemical spill releasing toxic or corrosive chemical (e.g., sulfuric acid)	Houston, spring season during rush hour

Source: Based on State of Texas 2013.[29(p76)]

Arguably, as Texas is the state with the most presidential disaster declarations, and as Galveston County has the most repetitive loss payments from disasters on a per-capita basis, Galveston County is the county most vulnerable to disasters in the most vulnerable state in United States.

Following the protocols of the DMA of 2000, Houston and Galveston formed a council in cooperation with 85 local governments to develop a regional hazard mitigation plan. The plan, approved by FEMA in 2006, included more than 300 proposed mitigation projects. These included the following:

- Purchasing flood-prone properties
- Increasing the capacity of culverts
- Improving drainage
- Building tornado shelters
- Protecting shorelines

The Houston–Galveston plan listed 11 major natural and two potential man-made hazards of concern:

1. Coastal erosion
2. Dam or levee failure
3. Drought
4. Excessive heat
5. Flood
6. Hail
7. Hurricanes and tropical storms
8. Severe thunderstorms
9. Tornadoes
10. Wildfires
11. Winter storms
12. Toxic releases
13. Energy pipeline failure

This list overlaps the plan for the State of Texas, but not perfectly. Specifically, the top five in the Houston–Galveston study ranked 6, 7, 3, 10, and 1, respectively, for the state as a whole.

Tier 3: Galveston City Hazard Mitigation Plan—the Nuts-and-Bolts Level

If you visit Galveston Island, we hope you will have time to see the striking memorial for the victims of the 1900 storm that struck Galveston, the most deadly storm in the history of the United States. The memorial appears on the front cover of the 2010–2013 Texas Hazard Mitigation Report.[26] Sitting on a barrier island, the city's roughly 50,000 residents need to be concerned about gradual sea-level rise. At current rates of change, by 2100, sea levels in Galveston will be approximately two feet higher than in 2015.[30]

Water from tropical storms is not the only reason why the Houston–Galveston mitigation plan was not the final step in hazard mitigation planning for Galveston City. After Hurricane Ike in 2008, the city requested support to develop its own plan because of its location on a barrier island. It seemed obvious that Galveston City's priorities should be somewhat different from those of the state and the Houston–Galveston County region.

A good way of understanding variation within this region is to go on a hypothetical drive from Rice University in Houston to Galveston City along Route 45. Throughout this roughly 85-minute drive (about 53 miles) land use changes between upper-income residential (Friendswood) to high technology (Houston Space Center), farming, open space, and industrial. The driver also passes two airports (William Hobby and George Bush), which are about 24 miles (38 kilometers) apart.

Heading southeast, the terrain abruptly changes near La Marque. Off to the east is Texas City, a port city of about 45,000 residents and a massive petroleum refining and petrochemical manufacturing complex. In 1947, a ship carrying ammonium nitrate exploded in Texas City. The explosion destroyed the facility, caused two additional ships to explode, and set some of Texas City's oil tanks and refineries ablaze. In total, 600 people were killed and 5,000 more were injured. In Galveston, 14 miles from Texas City, people were thrown to the ground. Texas City has suffered other hazard events, as well. These include Hurricane Carla in 1961, a large BP oil explosion in 2005, and Hurricane Ike in 2008. Luckily, the long dike levee system built around Texas City after Hurricane Carla limited the impact of the surge from Hurricane Ike. While the area was swamped, the dike pumps and other engineered systems saved Texas City from complete devastation. In 2016, the city remains only about 10 feet above sea level, which puts it at serious risk from storms, floods, and erosion. The combination of Texas City's massive petrochemical complex and its accompanying port facilities raises the economic and environmental health stakes for risk managers.

Leaving Texas City and driving west again and then south, it takes about 20 minutes to drive 14 miles to Galveston. Crossing Galveston Bay via a bridge on Route 45 into the city, abandoned lots abound. On September 28, 2011, the PBS news hour aired a feature "Galveston: the Mother of all U.S. Natural Disasters."[31] Jason Kane explained how the city tangled with two of the biggest storms in hurricane history—Ike and Carla—but actually focused on the massive hurricane in 1900. The editors used photography to cleverly pair images of what Galveston looked like immediately after the storm of 1900 and what it looked like in 2011. Indeed, Galveston had been a boomtown of 37,000 persons in 1900, known as the "Wall Street of the Southwest."

It served as a major deep-water port and was the first town in Texas to have telephone and electricity service—that is, until September 8, 1900. On that date, a hurricane with 140-mile-per-hour winds hit the town, sending a 15-foot-high storm surge over the 8.7-foot seawall. The story and photos show that one-third of the city was reduced to broken-up timbers. Amidst the devastation were more than 6,000 dead bodies, along with dead animals and rotting fish. Clara Barton and the Red Cross arrived in Galveston and reported that many volunteers were pale and ill as a result of what they saw.

The PBS show emphasized that Galveston built a 17-foot (5.2-meter) seawall and razed over 2,000 buildings to reduce their vulnerability. Nevertheless, Hurricanes Carla and Ike destroyed major parts of Galveston City in 1961 and 2008, respectively. The story concludes by characterizing the community as able to overcome these kinds of tragedies with toughness and grit.

Galveston's land use is diverse, although more than half of the land claimed as part of the city is underwater and unusable. Removing the portion of the city that is underwater, five land uses dominate:

1. Farms, ranches, and other agriculture-related land uses (51%)
2. Single-family residential (15%)
3. Vacant (8%)
4. Roads (7%)
5. Commercial (5%)[32]

The amount of agricultural and vacant land is unusual for a U.S. city but is a product of Galveston's location and history. A relatively small amount of land is devoted to university complexes, banks, and other financial institutions, but these are critical to the city and the mitigation planning process. Galveston City was a port for Mexico before the United States took over the land in 1835. It became a commercial center in the 19th century and has six historic districts with many Victorian and other homes on the National Register of Historic places. Galveston has a University of Texas Medical Branch as well as several other colleges, and it continues to have a large tourism industry including serving as a terminal for cruise lines. Banking and insurance companies started in Galveston in the 1840s continue to operate there today.

Population is a second source of Galveston's diversity. The U.S. Census Bureau's Factfinder provided some metrics that allow us to compare Galveston City's population vulnerability metrics to its neighbors and the State of Texas as a whole (Table 6.4).

The table shows that Galveston City's vulnerability is relatively high compared with the other three communities near it along Route 45, but not markedly so. In fact, the vulnerability index for U.S. counties for the years 2006 to 2010 showed that all of the Texas counties bordering on Mexico and many near the New Mexico border were among the top 20 percent in vulnerability to environmental hazards. Many were

Table 6.4. Demographic Indicators of Vulnerability for Galveston City, Nearby Communities, and the State of Texas

Metric	Galveston City	Friendswood	La Marque	Texas City	State of Texas
Population 65+ years old, July 1, 2010	13.6%	11.7%	13.8%	12.9%	10.3%
Population less than 5 years old, July 1, 2010	5.9%	5.2%	7.3%	7.5%	7.7%
Language other than English spoken at home, 2010-2014	28.0%	12.7%	17.9%	17.6%	34.9%
Population with a disability under the age of 65 years, 2010-2014	9.9%	4.4%	13.6%	13.2%	8.2%
Persons without health insurance, 2010-2014	27.1%	9.2%	27.0%	23.7%	21.3%
Persons in poverty 2010	23.7%	5.2%	19.2%	20.1%	17.2%

Source: Based on data from the U.S. Census Bureau.[33]

more vulnerable from a social perspective than those in the Houston–Galveston area.[30]

Galveston City Hazard Mitigation Plan

The city's risk assessment is critical so that the highest vulnerabilities are identified and risk managers can allocate resources to address them. If they do not, the risk mitigation process will be less effective at protecting human health, the environment, and assets than it could be. The City of Galveston's plan, especially its risk-assessment methodology, is good to review because it was prepared for a relatively small city and the process can be replicated in many other places.

The city organized a Hazard Mitigation Planning Stakeholder Committee (HMPSC) representing a variety of different interest groups in the municipality. As required by FEMA, the HMPSC developed goals. These goals are paraphrased here:

- Improve education and outreach efforts to the public, elected officials, municipal employees, and local businesses regarding potential impacts of hazards and methods to reduce these impacts.
- Improve opportunities at the municipal level to plan and implement hazard mitigation plans, especially by forming partnerships with universities and private organizations and by using geographic information systems and other tools (statistical methods, risk assessment, loss assessment).
- Develop hazard mitigation policies and programs to reduce impacts of natural and human hazards on people and property.
- Identify and implement hazard mitigation projects.

These four goals are truly generic and would apply to the vast majority of jurisdictions in the United States. The goals were supported by six general objectives oriented toward reducing economic consequences:

1. Improve public education about actions in which they can engage to reduce deaths, injuries, and property damage.
2. Obtain, update, and maintain data about vulnerabilities of the critical facilities and historical assets.
3. Seek methods to reduce to National Flood Insurance Program claims.
4. Examine methods to manage development to keep people and property out of harm's way.
5. Engage in opportunities to mitigate repetitive loss and severe repetitive loss properties.
6. Seek opportunities to increase participation and compliance with National Flood Insurance Programs and the Community Rating Systems.

The HMPSC listed some general policies, projects, and programs to advance these objectives:

1. Install emergency generators.
2. Retrofit and harden existing facilities.
3. Upgrade flood control infrastructure.
4. Build a safe room (from wind, weather, and other disasters).
5. Protect critical systems needed for mitigation.
6. Focus on public education.
7. Install warning systems.

Galveston City's mostly qualitative risk assessment was produced without a massive amount of resources. The HMPSC relied primarily on the local knowledge and experience of its committee members and city staff; studies conducted by or for the city; existing city plans; and studies, reports, and plans produced by federal, state, and local agencies. Indeed, if the process remains transparent with input solicited from stakeholders who represent the breadth of the community, their risk mitigation plan has a good chance of succeeding.

It appears that the analysts creating the risk mitigation plan for Galveston used the damages caused by Hurricane Ike to assess the economic costs and benefits of their mitigation ideas. Table 6.5 provides their risk definitions.

The risk analysts aggregated 28 hazards of concern into 14 categories, assessing five of the categories to pose low risk: (1) a biological event, (2) coastal subsidence, (3) drought, (4) lightning, and (5) tsunami. Table 6.6 lists the assessed risk for the remaining nine categories of hazards of concern.

Each of these rankings (high to low) was accompanied by a discussion that explained the ranking decision. The risk assessment clearly focused on flooding, followed by

Table 6.5. Definitions of Risk Assessment Terminology Used in the Galveston City, Texas, Report

Term	Potential Impact to Lives, Safety, and Livelihood	Potential Impact to Buildings and Critical Facilities	Potential Impact to Infrastructure
Low	Some injuries possible but unlikely	• Cosmetic damages to structures • Loss of function for less than one day	Some roads and/or bridges temporarily not useable
Moderate	Injuries expected, some deaths possible	• Some structural damages • Loss of function for one to two days	• Roads and/or bridge closures • Power and utility loss
High	Several deaths expected	Some structures irreparably damaged loss of function for three to five days	• Long-term road and/or bridge closures • Long-term power and utility loss

Source: Based on data from City of Galveston 2011.[30]

extreme wind and wildfire or urban fire. These three hazard risks, as well as coastal erosion and hazardous materials incidents, were deemed to be of sufficient concern to warrant what the report calls a "quantitative risk assessment" (see Chapter 8 for a discussion of one done at a former nuclear weapons site). We have selected one of these risks for further discussion—extreme wind risks from severe thunderstorms, straight line winds, tropical systems or hurricanes, and tornadoes.

The first federally declared disaster of 12 caused by extreme wind in Galveston was in 1961. The second occurred in 1998 and 10 more followed between 1998 and 2008. Eight of the 12 extreme wind disasters were caused by hurricanes and the remaining four were

Table 6.6. Results of Qualitative Risk Assessment: Galveston City, 2011

Hazard	Potential Impact to People's Lives, Safety, and Livelihood	Potential Impact to Buildings or Critical Facilities	Potential Impact to Infrastructure
Extreme wind	High	High	High
Flooding	Moderate	High	High
Terrorism	Moderate/High	Moderate/High	Moderate/High
Sea level rise	Low	Moderate	Moderate
Environmental disaster	Moderate/High	Low	Low
Coastal erosion	Low	Moderate	Moderate
Wildfire or urban fire	Moderate	High	Low
Coastal retreat	Low	Low/Moderate	Moderate
Hazardous materials incident (fixed site and transport)	Low/Moderate	Low/Moderate	Low/Moderate

Source: Based on data from City of Galveston 2011.[30]

Table 6.7. Extreme Wind Recurrence Intervals: Galveston City, Texas, Risk Assessment

Event Frequency, Years	Average Anticipated Wind Speed	Maximum Anticipated Wind Speed
10	67	74
20	86	97
50	111	116
100	124	125
200	133	134
500	144	149
1000	151	155

Source: Based on data from City of Galveston 2011.[30]

caused by tropical storms and a severe storm. This information, along with other data, was used to estimate the likelihood of wind speeds at specific recurrence intervals. For example, a 10-year average anticipated wind speed was estimated to be 67 miles per hour. The less probable events have increasingly higher wind speeds as shown in Table 6.7.

The Galveston report displays areas likely to be hit by various hurricane storm tracks, which gives the user a visual impression of where wind events would occur. Using a version of HAZUS, an economic model (see Chapter 9 for discussion of economic impact models), analysts estimated that the city and its population can expect property losses of about $32 million, or 0.8 percent of total asset values per year. About 62 percent of this loss would be in residential structures and another 12 percent in commercial structures.

Another way of looking at vulnerability was to examine 71 critical facilities in the city. During a 100-year hurricane (1 in 100 chance of occurring in a given year), the analysts estimated that with winds averaging 124 miles per hour, three of the 71 critical facilities would experience a total loss of function and the other 68 would suffer a partial loss. A 500-year wind event (1 in 500 chance of occurring in a given year) averaging 144 miles per hour was expected to cause all 71 critical facilities to experience a total loss of function. This illustrates the potential severity of a low-probability but high-consequence event such as wind striking a barrier island containing a city that is 28 miles long and between 0.5 and 2.5 miles wide, even if the barrier island is protected by a 10-mile-long seawall that is 17 feet high and 16 feet thick.

Overall, the list of highest priorities for Galveston City certainly aligns with the state priorities and the Houston–Galveston area ones. Floods are among the highest priority across all three, followed by wildfires, coastal erosion, and wind storms.

The bottom line for hazard mitigation planning is to pick projects that address the goals and objectives and have the capability to implement the plan. Galveston's year-2014 progress report[32] allows us to review the risk mitigation priorities, their progress, and any modifications. Table 6.8 lists selective projects in the context of the four broad city hazard mitigation goals presented earlier. Far more data are presented in the report. Sometimes projects have been deferred due to a lack of funding or a need to move money to address the aftermath of

Table 6.8. Selected Hazard Mitigation Projects for Galveston City, Texas, in the Context of Four Major Goals

Goal	Status	Estimated Cost	Comment	Priority
Number 1: Public Education				
Educate residents and visitors.	Ongoing	$2,000	Town hall meeting, local television, newspapers, Web site, Facebook, Twitter	High
Use Internet to provide information about preparation for natural disasters.	Ongoing	$21,000	Use Web site, Facebook, and Twitter	High
Hold town meeting before hurricane season.	Ongoing	$2,000	Town meeting	High
Purchase and distribute NOAA all-hazard radios to public facilities, schools, day care, medical facilities, critical facilities, and large public gathering places.	Ongoing	$100 per unit	Located in key places	High
Number 2: Partnering and Using Tools				
Work with NOAA and other agencies to study sea-level rise in Galveston.	New, deferred	$5,000+		Moderate
Develop sustainability plan implementation.	Ongoing, underway	$50,000	Completed in 2013	Moderate
Digitize paper records for preservation of the information after a disaster rather than lose the history of procedures and operations.	Underway	$5,000+	Ongoing	Moderate
Develop detailed inventory of critical facilities.	New	$5,000	Applies to existing and future development	High
Number 3: Develop Hazard Mitigation Policies and Programs				
Consider joining the National Flood Insurance Program's community rating system.	Existing, ongoing	$10,000	Membership and successful completion leads to lower costs for community	Moderate
Increase cadre of floodplain managers through training and certification.	New	$10,000	Increased by four and will continue to increase	Moderate
Identify repetitive loss properties for mitigation.	Completed	Unknown	Action completed	
Restore destroyed dune systems.	Ongoing	Unknown	Ongoing in aftermath of Hurricane Ike	Moderate

(Continued)

Table 6.8. (Continued)

Goal	Status	Estimated Cost	Comment	Priority
Number 4: Identify and Implement Projects				
Identify, elevate, or acquire repetitive-loss properties.	Existing, modified, deferred	$50,000+ loss per property	Applies to existing structures	High
Remove debris and physical threats to public and property.	Completed	Unknown	Action completed	High
Elevate coastal roads.	Existing, modified, deferred	Unknown	Partially completed	High
Improve drainage projects and better maintenance.	Ongoing	Unknown	Existing and future drainage systems	High
Elevate structures at risk of flooding.	Ongoing	$50,000–$100,000+ loss per property	Existing structures, new structures must meet new codes	High
Purchase test equipment for local cable channel.	Completed	$20,000		High
Identify and purchase equipment and vehicles.	Existing, ongoing, modified	$750,000	Ongoing replacement and upgrade partly supported by FEMA	High
Harden facility and improve security at water pumping station.	Completed	$600,000	Completed in 2011	Moderate
Harden facility and improve security at unmanned municipal utility facilities.	Existing, underway	$2.5 million	Design underway	Moderate
Mitigate and harden substantially damaged historic and other structures.	Existing, ongoing, modified	$50,000+ loss per property	Applied to existing and future structures	Moderate
Design and construct a safe room to house emergency personnel who must remain on the island during evacuations.	Existing, ongoing	$10–$15 million	Applied for and under investigation	Moderate
Increase native canopy by tree planting in public rights of way to reduce heat island effect.	Existing, ongoing	$500,000	Applies to existing and future development	Moderate
Develop and implement early detection system for hazardous materials incidents, leaks, and accidents.	Existing, modified, ongoing	$25,000+	Private funding	Moderate
Develop and implement stormwater drainage system improvements.	Existing, deferred	$250 million	Existing and new development	Moderate

Source: Based on City of Galveston 2014.[32]

Note: FEMA=Federal Emergency Management Agency; NOAA=National Oceanic and Atmospheric Administration.

an event such as Hurricane Ike. The 26 projects listed represent about half of the ideas in the report. The breadth is impressive, and the costs range from $2,000 for an annual meeting to $250 million for rebuilding the city's drainage system. The HMPSC can find resources to pay for some of the smaller projects, but a small city of fewer than 50,000 will need assistance from FEMA and other parties for larger ones. For purposes of the reader, the menu of projects is illustrative of risk management options in wind- and flood-prone areas.

Although Galveston is a small city with a great deal of experience at managing hazards, it does not have the resources of Houston, Austin, San Antonio, Dallas, Fort Worth, and other much larger Texas cities. To get a sense of its capabilities, we reviewed the capability assessment section of its 2011 plan, which is centered on a 2010 survey of the following attributes:

- Staff, personnel, and technical capability
- Knowledge of FEMA's programs
- Current efforts
- Coordination
- Land use and associated regulations
- Floodplain management
- Building code implementation
- Capital improvement
- Local conservation programs
- Fiscal, administrative, and regulatory capacity

With the caveat that the authors have not personally interviewed the local hazard mitigation team, this city seems far more capable than others of similar size. Indeed, the vast majority of cities the size of Galveston are part of larger county and regional plans, as was Galveston City until Hurricane Ike. Clearly, the city has had support from FEMA, the State of Texas, and the Houston–Galveston region. It will need more to address the large, expensive physical projects that are part of its portfolio of planned mitigation projects. The Galveston case study leads us to recall the proverb, "Necessity is the mother of invention."

Final Thoughts

Analysis of demographic data, including statistical analysis and mapping, are routine in public health and planning. Applying these resources to keep people and assets out of harm's way is necessary as the marketplace makes decisions without accounting for vulnerability and possible impacts—consequences that cause injuries and destroy lives and assets. Many of our younger students cannot understand how some structures were allowed to be placed in high-risk locations. Were we to rewind the clock and start de novo, we suspect that even developers would stop the clock and rethink their ideas.

The hazard mitigation planning mechanism removes the opportunity for local officials to ignore the consequences of siting decisions. Public health and planning practitioners should familiarize themselves with their state and local hazard mitigation plans and assess how they may need to adjust their existing land use plans to prevent serious consequences. They may also need to upgrade local codes to harden facilities and make them more resilient. In some cases, it makes no sense to allow new facilities, such as the assisted living facility proposed in the first paragraph, to be located in a vulnerable area. It often makes sense to require major investments to upgrade existing facilities and even to harden new ones.

Every hazard mitigation plan is grounded in and, in most cases, uses every tool described and illustrated in this book. Hazard mitigation planning and implementation should be a major directive of every public health and planning official practicing at the local scale. It makes no sense to pretend otherwise.

References

1. Cutter SL, Boruff BJ, Shirley WL. Social vulnerability to environmental hazards. *Soc Sci Q*. 2003;84(2):242–261.

2. Hazards and Vulnerability Research Institute. Social Vulnerability Index for the United States 2006–10. Available at: http://artsandsciences.sc.edu/geog/hvri/sovi®-0. Accessed March 7, 2017.

3. Greenberg M. Keep out? Housing, social and physicial environments of neighborhoods bordering major cities and their suburbs. In: Hammond E, Noyes A, eds. *Housing: Socioeconomic, Availability and Development Issues*. New York, NY: Nova Publishers; 2009:87–100.

4. Pflicke K, Greenberg M, Whytlaw J, Herb J, Kaplan M. Populations vulnerable to climate change in New Jersey: update of a statistical analysis. Rutgers University, New Jersey Climate Change Depository. 2015. Available at: https://rucore.libraries.rutgers.edu/rutgers-lib/46837. Accessed March 8, 2017.

5. Kraak M-J, Ormeling F. *Cartography: Visualization of Geospatial Data*. 3rd ed. New York, NY: Routledge; 2013.

6. Tyner J. *The World of Maps*. New York, NY: Guilford Press; 2015.

7. Birkland TA. *Lessons of Disaster: Policy Change After Catastrophic Events*. Washington, DC: Georgetown University Press; 2006.

8. *Multi-Hazard Mitigation Planning Guidance Under the Disaster Mitigation Act of 2000*. Washington, DC: Federal Emergency Management Agency; 2008.

9. Burby RJ, Beatley T, Berke PR, et al. Unleashing the power of planning to create disaster-resistant communities. *J Am Plan Assoc*. 1999;65(3):247–258.

10. Godschalk D, Beatley T, Berke P, Brower D, Kaiser EJ. *Natural Hazard Mitigation: Recasting Disaster Policy and Planning*. Washington, DC: Island Press; 1999.

11. Mazmanian DA. The three epochs of the environmental movement. In: Mazmanian DA, Kraft ME, eds. *Toward Sustainable Communities: Transition and Transformations in Environmental Policy*. Cambridge, MA: MIT Press; 2009:3–41.

12. Mileti D. *Disasters by Design: A Reassessment of Natural Hazards in the United States*. Washington, DC: Joseph Henry Press; 1999.

13. Nolon JR. Climate change and sustainable development: the quest for green communities, Part II. *Plan Environ Law*. 2009;61(11):3–15.

14. Smith G. Planning for sustainable and disaster resilient communities. In: Pine J, ed. *Hazard Analysis*. Washington, DC: Taylor & Francis; 2008:221–247.

15. Federal Emergency Management Agency. Hazard mitigation planning. Available at: http://www.fema.gov/hazard-mitigation-planning. Accessed March 7, 2017.

16. Smith G. A Review of the United States Disaster Assistance Framework: Planning for Recovery. 2010. Available at: http://doctorflood.rice.edu/sspeed/downloads/May26_2010/16.%20 Gavin%20Smith%20-%20Coastal%20Symposium.pdf. Accessed August 20, 2016.

17. Berke P, Godschalk D. Searching for the good plan: a meta-analysis of plan quality studies. *J Plan Lit*. 2009;23(3):227–240.

18. Berke P, Backhurst M, Day M, et al. What makes plan implementation successful? An evaluation of local plans and implementation practices in New Zealand. *Environ Plan B Plan Des*. 2006;33(4):581–600.

19. Brody S, Highfield W. Planning at the urban fringe: an examination of the factors influencing nonconforming development patterns in southern Florida. *Environ Plan*. 2006;33(1):75–96.

20. Dalton L, Burby R. Mandates, plans, and planners: building local commitment to development management. *J Am Plan Assoc*. 1994;60(4):444–461.

21. Deyle R, Chapin T, Baker E. The proof of the planning is in the platting: an evaluation of Florida's hurricane exposure mitigation planning mandate. *J Am Plan Assoc*. 2008;74(3):349–370.

22. Nelson A, French S. Plan quality and mitigating damage from natural disasters: a case study of the Northridge earthquake with planning policy considerations. *J Am Plan Assoc*. 2002;68(2):94–207.

23. Whiteman D. 10 states most at risk for major disasters. Bankrate. 2014. Available at: http://www.bankrate.com/finance/weather/natural-disasters/states-most-at-risk-for-major-disasters-1.aspx. Accessed March 7, 2017.

24. Freedman A. Top 5 most vulnerable US cities to hurricanes. Climate Central. June 6, 2012. Available at: http://www.climatecentral.org/news/top-5-most-vulnerable-us-cities-to-hurricanes. Accessed March 7, 2017.

25. Pickles K. From hurricanes and flooding to wildfires and earthquakes: the top 10 US cities most at risk of natural disaster—and all but one are in the South. September 24, 2015. *Daily Mail*. Available at: http://www.dailymail.co.uk/news/article-3247407/From-hurricanes-flooding-wildfires-earthquakes-10-cities-risk-natural-disasters-one-South.html. Accessed March 7, 2017.

26. State of Texas Hazard Mitigation Plan 2010–2013. 2010. Available at: https://www.txdps.state.tx.us/dem/documents/txHazMitPlan.pdf. Accessed August 20, 2016.

27. United States and Texas Populations 1850–2015. 2016. Texas State Library and Archives Commission. Available at: https://www.tsl.texas.gov/ref/abouttx/census.html. Accessed March 7, 2017.

28. Berke P, Smith G, Lyles W. Planning for resiliency: evaluation of state hazard mitigation plans under the Disaster Mitigation Act. *Nat Hazards Rev*. 2012;13(2):139–149.

29. State of Texas Hazard Mitigation Plan: 2013 Update. 2013. Available at: http://txdps.state.tx.us/dem/Mitigation/txHazMitPlan.pdf. Accessed August 20, 2016.

30. City of Galveston. Hazard Mitigation Plan. 2012. Available at: http://galvestontx.gov/DocumentCenter/Home/View/2277. Accessed March 7, 2017.

31. Kane J. Galveston: the mother of all US natural disasters. PBS Newshour. September 28, 2011. Available at: http://www.pbs.org/newshour/rundown/galveston-the-mother-of-all-us-natural-disasters. Accessed March 7, 2017.

32. *City of Galveston Hazard Mitigation Plan, Annual Report, 2014 Progress Report.* Galveston, TX: City of Galveston Office of Emergency Management; 2014.

33. US Census Bureau. 2010 census interactive population search: Galveston City, Texas. Available at: https://www.census.gov/2010census/popmap/ipmtext.php?fl=48. Accessed August 2, 2017.

7

MANAGING LEGAL AND MORAL OBLIGATIONS

The context for this chapter is that your state and/or the federal government have imposed a program on your locality, or your local government has chosen to respond to a moral commitment. We highlight tools and processes that are important when the need is to help or house abused women and children, alcohol and other drug abusers, the food insecure, persons who are homeless, stressed veterans, those recently released from incarceration, or new immigrants.

Each of these vulnerable populations has somewhat different needs. Each will engender different reactions from the community because of individual and collective values, perceptions, and beliefs, as well as positions taken by elected officials. The bottom line is that legal and moral obligations can be wonderful opportunities and they can lead to painful community-changing disputes.[1] Tools described elsewhere in this book, such as checklists, outreach and dissemination tools, health impact assessments (HIAs), hazard mapping, environmental assessment, planning and design charrettes, and environmental management all apply to these challenges. However, in addition to these, we picked the following three to highlight in this chapter because of the deep social and political content of meeting moral obligations:

1. Social network analysis
2. Environmental justice assessment
3. Political process assessment

We demonstrate these tools and others with two California cases. One is about building an integrated program for homeless veterans with physical and mental health and employment challenges. The second focuses on providing access to healthy food for poor people.

These challenging missions require that public health and planning officials answer three questions:

1. What are the goals of the group(s) leading the project (which may or may not be your group)? Social network analysis will help answer this question.
2. Are the goals appropriate to the people in your area? Social and environmental justice assessments focus on answering this question.

3. How can the project be designed, implemented, and communicated to help decision-makers understand the project? Political process assessment should answer this question.

To be clear, it is not our intention to turn every planner and health official into a sociologist, political scientist, or social engineer. As in the other case study chapters, it is to provide readers with analytical and process tools that will help them make better decisions.

Social Network Analysis

Social network analysis, initially developed in the 1930s, focuses on identifying networks of interacting people. Social analysts distinguish between nodes (people and organizations) and links (meetings, phone calls, and other communication paths) that connect the nodes and the ideas they created.[2-5] Readers who have worked with water, sewer, rail, road, and other transportation networks will recognize that these terms emanate from graph theory; they are widely used in infrastructure engineering. For example, the first author's PhD thesis in the late 1960s was about moving water from reservoirs, lakes, and other nodes that had excess water despite a drought, to places that were running out of water. The links were a network of pipes, pumps, and other engineered structures that delivered fresh water from the sources to the areas of demand.

During the 1970s, opportunities to understand social networks substantially increased with the advent of high-speed computers. Studies of social networks have markedly increased with the introduction of Facebook, Twitter, and other electronic-based social media. The local library, town hall, local gazette, and religious institution are still part of the social network, but increasingly electronic transmissions are where the bulk of communications take place. For example, Mislove and colleagues[3] analyzed multiple online social networks such as Orkut, YouTube, and Flickr, observing that the typical network can be divided into strong and weak members. About 10 percent of the strong members constitute the core (nodes), which receives more than half the messages (links). The strong members are popular and trusted; they post their goals, history, and much of their strategy on the Web. They may maintain a blog or other Web site, comment often on a social Web site, or otherwise remain linked. If you want to learn more about a particular social network, you can join the group Web site or work with someone who has.

Social network analysis is important because social networks are increasingly at the heart of efforts to diffuse public health and planning ideas and principles. For example, Ennett and colleagues[6] found that runaway and homeless youth with a social network, even a small one, were much less likely to engage in dangerous behaviors involving alcohol, drugs, and sex compared with those who were socially isolated. This may indicate to those planning programs for this cohort that linking to various types of social media will help their organization with effective outreach.

Sometimes the results of social network analysis may be contradictory. Consider, for example, the relationship of healthy eating with food networks. Christakis and Fowler[7] reported that social networks, along with environmental conditions, helped spread the problem of obesity across the United States. By contrast, Cohen-Cole and Fletcher[8] reanalyzed the same data and found that social networks were not a contributor. We are not suggesting that planners and public health officials purchase and learn to use social network analysis software. However, a good literature review will aid them in figuring out which social networks to investigate for their purposes.

As an example, Friedman's[9] poignant case report of a 38-year-old veteran illustrates the challenge of assisting soldiers that had participated in combat. This particular veteran was married with two children and was an auto salesman before his National Guard Unit went to Iraq. While on duty, he killed people, watched his friends get killed, and watched Iraqi women and children get killed. In his own words, "Life has become a terrible burden." He reported that he sometimes thinks everyone would be better off if he had not survived his tour in Iraq. How can your community help veterans struggling with various types of problems? Pietrzak and colleagues[10] found that strong support from a dedicated veterans' unit and postdeployment social support were associated with the decreased likelihood of posttraumatic stress disorder (PTSD) and depression. Boscarino[11] observed that those who were in combat were more likely to exhibit PTSD, anxiety, and depression than were veterans who had not seen combat. Participating in a local social support group reduced many self-destructive behaviors for these veterans, with the exception of drug abuse. Mares et al.[12] found that a social network and permanent housing, along with treatment, are essential for traumatized veterans. Perhaps your local community can help organize a social support group or provide referral services for veterans?

The literature offers an equally strong set of cases for the value of social networks in addressing food security. For example, Whatmore and Thorne[13] discuss food pantries as an interconnected set of social and organizational networks. Hamelin and colleagues[14] consider the food security problem to be so extensive that they fully expect a continually expanding network of socially and politically organized food pantries to be the new normal. Despite the growth of food pantries and organized food networks, Ahluwalia et al.[15] note that people want to rely on families first, only reluctantly turning to friends and then even more reluctantly to more distant parts of their social networks. In Hartford, Connecticut, Dhokarh and colleagues[16] found that lack of acculturation and lack of social networks exacerbate food insecurity among Puerto Rican families. In an overarching critique, Campbell[17] points to a rapidly growing network designed to respond to food insecurity, noting that the effort brings out some of the best and worst practices in planning and public health. To avoid serious local and institutional conflicts, she recommends building mutually agreed upon plans of action for food security in a community by using networks of motivated individuals.

Overall, a basic understanding of social networks is essential to understand the context for legally mandated and moral and social issues that require a response from health and planning officials. Specifically, it is vitally important to know the history of the issue, the key groups (nodes) to engage, their objectives, and strategies. These can normally be found on the Web, at local meetings, and with selected phone calls.

Social and Environmental Justice

In the United States, the civil rights movement of the 1960s merged into the environmental justice movement two decades later. The U.S. Environmental Protection Agency's (EPA's) legal definition of environmental justice is "the fair treatment and meaningful involvement of all people regardless of race, color, national origin, or income, with respect to the development, implementation, and enforcement of environmental laws, regulations and policies."[18] In practice, that definition does not include all non-white populations, all ages, and all persons with assorted disabilities and health problems, unless they are poor. This definition was the product of the late 20th century and has not been altered to be more inclusive.

We start here with two tools: the U.S. Census Bureau data and EJSCREEN, free resources that are linked. The U.S. Census Bureau publishes data at the national, state, county, and local government levels. These data are crucial to understanding the geography of human health and safety risk (see Chapter 6 for a discussion of how to access census data).

EJSCREEN[19] is a tool developed by the EPA in 2014. The agency's goals were to have a nationally consistent tool that would allow the agency and interested individuals to compare environmental justice–related issues across all of the states. One set of indicators is potential hazard exposures: (1) air toxics cancer risk, (2) air toxics respiratory hazards, and (3) air toxics neurodevelopment hazards. At this time, all of these data are not available for every location.

A second set of potential hazard exposure indicators includes the following:

- Level of diesel particulate matter in the air ($\mu g/m^3$)
- Annual average of fine particulate matter (PM 2.5) in the air ($\mu g/m^3$)
- Ozone summer seasonal average of daily maximum eight-hour concentration in the air (ppb)
- Lead paint (percentage of housing units built before 1960 is used as a surrogate)

The third set of potential hazard exposure indicators listed by EPA is as follows:

- Traffic and volume, calculated as average annual daily traffic at major roads within 500 meters, divided by distance in meters

- Proximity to major direct dischargers to water, calculated as count of major direct water discharge facilities within 5 kilometers (or nearest one beyond 5 kilometers), each divided by distance in kilometers
- Proximity to Superfund sites or National Priority List (NPL) sites, calculated as count of proposed and listed NPL sites within 5 kilometers (or nearest one beyond 5 kilometers), each divided by distance in kilometers
- Proximity to potential chemical accident management plan or risk management plan (RMP) facilities, calculated as count of RMP facilities within 5 kilometers (or nearest one beyond 5 kilometers), each divided by distance in kilometers
- Proximity to hazardous waste management facilities or treatment storage and disposal facilities (TSDFs), calculated count of TSDFs within 5 kilometers (or nearest one beyond 5 kilometers), each divided by distance in kilometers

EJSCREEN allows the user to query a city, town, and specific area by name, census tract code, or even latitude and longitude. The user simply draws a polygon or drops an electronic pin where a circle of a particular radius is created around a site of interest. EJSCREEN sends back output allowing the user to compare the study area with the state as a whole and the nation. Results appear in graphs and tables using a scale of 0 (lowest) to 100 (highest). Hence, a score of 50 means that the area is average.

To illustrate the use of EJSCREEN, we located the neighborhood in Flint, Michigan, that was found to have a high drinking water lead burden.[20] The 1-mile radius around the neighborhood in Flint scored 80 to 90 percent in PM 2.5, ozone, lead paint risk, NPL proximity, and TSDF proximity compared with the State of Michigan as a whole. It also had slightly higher traffic proximity and water discharge proximity than did the entire state. In other words, the area of Flint found to have high levels of lead in its drinking water would be among the top 20 percent in the United States with regard to environmental exposures from contaminated air and potential industrial hazards.

Demographically, the population in the 1-mile radius area around the Flint neighborhood with the highest lead exposures is 58 percent black and 11 percent other minorities. EJSCREEN reports that 54 percent of the population had a household income of less than $25,000 per year during the period 2008 to 2012, and 63 percent were renting their residence. This area of Flint presents the profile of a neighborhood with serious social and environmental justice challenges, but not the worst that the authors have seen (see the case study of South Los Angeles later in this chapter).

Overall, it takes about 45 minutes to read and apply the EJSCREEN instructions. We recommend that you test it on the place where you live or work, or have lived or worked in the past. It is easy to use and a helpful screening tool, but it is not without limitations. For instance, we do not know what an 80 to 90 percent score in EJSCREEN means with regard to human health risk. Nor does a low score such as 10 to 20 percent imply no risk to human health and safety. Risk assessment (Chapter 8) is required to help answer those questions.

Political Process Assessment

Understanding processes that lead to the emergence, spread, and sometimes decline of major social movements can be critical to making effective decisions. Political process assessment requires answering three questions:

1. What grievances motivated members of the group to organize?
2. Have they built an organization(s) with financial, political, social, media, and other supporters?
3. What vulnerabilities in the existing political and social systems engendered the emergence of the issue? For example, has the existing political and economic leadership lost some control of its constituents, allowing new challenges to emerge? A war, a violent event, or other incidents that weaken control often trigger an opportunity for successful challenge of existing rules, procedures, and processes.

The civil rights movement in the United States, which began in the early 20th century, is probably the best known illustration.[21-31] Black Americans have had a long list of grievances from the days of the first importation of slaves. These have included the inability to vote, serve on juries, attend schools with white counterparts, purchase a house or rent an apartment in any neighborhood, and feel safe in the street and in their residences, among others.

The black community formed the National Association for the Advancement of Colored People (NAACP) in 1909 and the National Urban League in 1911.[24,25] The groups organized and used lawsuits to attack the idea of separate-but-equal schools. With some success, the community resorted to mass nonviolent protests in the form of sit-ins, boycotts, marches, and freedom rides that brought out large numbers of people.[21-23,26-30]

Whites joined some of these, as did organizations, black-owned businesses, and a variety of religious institutions. When the governor of Arkansas called out the National Guard to prevent African American students from entering a high school in Little Rock, Arkansas, President Eisenhower told them to return to their quarters and sent in the members of the 101st Airborne to protect the students. At every step, there was resistance, but the organization was growing and gaining allies, such as Hubert Humphrey and Lyndon Johnson, and eventually Robert Kennedy and John F. Kennedy.[27,28] Key American labor leaders including Walter Reuther strongly supported the movement, as did a large segment of the American Jewish community.

The U.S. power structure that opposed equal rights was vulnerable to legal challenges. For example, *Brown v. Board of Education* undermined the principle of keeping blacks in segregated all-black schools.[24-29] The United States was markedly vulnerable at the international scale to charges that the country that was preaching democracy to other nations did not provide it to all its citizens.[30] The Ku Klux Klan's efforts to use physical intimidation and violence outraged many Americans.

U.S. businesses in some locations were vulnerable to boycotts and sit-ins and had to ease or eliminate their restrictions to survive. Public universities in Mississippi, Alabama, and several other states had prevented blacks from enrolling but, after a decade or more of these practices, they failed because of continuing pressure to open universities to all citizens. Black World War II veterans often returned to segregation and other oppressive conditions that they had escaped during the war, especially after President Truman ordered desegregation of the armed forces.

There were galvanizing trigger events. Perhaps the most dramatic were associated with the civil unrest identified with the assassination of Dr. Martin Luther King, Jr., on April 4, 1968. However, the vulnerability of cities was demonstrated earlier with civil unrest in Harlem, New York City, in 1964; Watts, in Los Angeles, California, in 1965; and in Atlanta, Georgia; San Francisco, California; Baltimore, Maryland; Seattle, Washington; Cleveland, Ohio; Cincinnati, Ohio; Newark, New Jersey; and Detroit, Michigan, in 1966 to 1967. The media portrayed the events as a clash between police and black demonstrators and their white allies. The issues highlighted by the media were lack of representation in police forces and excess use of force. However, the issues were far more complicated, involving poor housing, poor education, and lack of job opportunities, among others. More than 100 U.S. cities experienced civil unrest in 1967. President Johnson created the National Advisory Commission on Civil Disorders (the Commission),[31] which clearly described the difficult position of black Americans. The Commission traced the history of efforts to make black lives both better and worse, as well as the immediate issues of the civil unrest. In essence, the landmark book put out by the Commission said that the United States was becoming more racially segregated, headed toward separate societies. After Dr. King's assassination in 1968, this vulnerability intensified across the United States at the local and neighborhood, as well as national and state, political levels.

The civil rights movement continues today, with every step having been documented, much of it addressing political and social processes. This information can be used to answer the three questions posed previously using the tools and process presented here. This information may be helpful to your own communities.

Case Study: Helping Returning Veterans

Some veterans experienced no problems after returning to the United States from a war zone. Others returned home disabled, some were emotionally distressed, and many just needed some help and time to adjust. Veterans' groups have reported that resentment and anger has been building because of the lack of support in the following areas:

- Health care, including mental health
- Housing, including finding and paying for a residence for the homeless

- Access to education
- Access and training for employment
- Family support
- Disability and death benefits

Federal Resources

The United States formally recognizes the importance of war veterans. For instance, Armistice Day was first celebrated in 1919, and it became a national holiday in 1938. Former four-star general and President of the United States Dwight Eisenhower was instrumental in changing the name to Veteran's Day, which is celebrated every November 11. Federal and state programs dedicated to helping veterans have also been created. The federal government's programs start with U.S. Department of Veterans Affairs (VA).

Veterans need a stable home environment before they can deal with issues of drug and other substance abuse, psychological trauma, and finding good employment. The VA's Housing Assistance program,[32] the U.S. Interagency Council on Homelessness,[33] and the U.S. Department of Housing and Urban Development Veterans Assistance program[34] have been working on finding housing for homeless veterans, including providing VA loans, rental assistance, and housing vouchers. The U.S. Department of Defense, VA, and Department of Labor sponsored the creation of a National Resource Directory[35] that can be used to find help from government, private, and not-for-profit agencies at different geographical levels across a wide range of services that veterans might need. Another interesting federal-scale option is the Joining Forces Initiative,[36] which seeks to partner with local governments to provide assistance to veterans and their families.

State Resources

Some states have programs dedicated to veterans. To determine what is available in your state, we suggest searching the Web. We live in New Jersey. Our state has an 18-page "New Jersey Veterans' Benefits Guide"[37] that includes the following:

- Medical benefits, insurance (e.g., eyeglasses, hearing aids, and dental care/health insurance)
- Health care for women veterans
- Obtaining a VA identification card
- Locations of veterans' centers in New Jersey, Pennsylvania, and New York, along with phone and email contact information
- Information for those concerned about PTSD

- Support services for veterans' families
- Housing, homeless, and home keeper programs
- Home loans, property tax benefits
- Employment, business opportunities
- Education and tuition benefits
- Vehicle registration
- Long-term-care nursing facilities managed by the New Jersey Department of Military VA
- Transportation programs
- Death, burial, and related benefits

The guide even includes an easy-to-remember phone number (1-888-8NJ-VETS). It appears that New Jersey has tried to provide information for veterans and their families in a readable format. A document such as this one is mirrored in every state, and it is worth consulting yours to understand the network of public and private organizations you can contact for your jurisdiction.

Not-for-Profit and Philanthropic Organizations

Table 7.1 lists some well-known nongovernmental organizations that provide support for veterans, starting with the American Legion and ending with the Vietnam Veterans of America. Some provide broad categories of assistance; others are more narrowly focused on housing.

In short, there is no shortage of groups and programs directed to assist veterans, and their objectives are almost always clearly defined on their Web site, even though some appear at first glance to offer duplicative services.

Veterans' Attributes

Should you be involved in a program that focuses or even partly includes veterans, it is prudent to visit the U.S. Census Bureau files and use EJSCREEN. The U.S. Census Bureau reports that there are about 22 million veterans in the United States, about 8 percent of the national population.[38] The racial/ethnic demographics of these veterans are as follows:

- White, non-Latino (80.2%)
- Black (11.0%)
- Hispanic/Latino (5.5%)
- Asian (1.2%)
- American Indian or Alaska Native (0.7%)

Table 7.1. Leading Veterans' Not-for-Profit and Philanthropic Organizations

Organization	Web Link	Main Objectives
American Legion	https://www.legion.org	Multiple services to veterans
American Veterans	http://www.amvets.org	Direct help to veterans
Disabled American Veterans	https://www.dav.org	Assistance to disabled veterans and public education
Habitat for Humanity	http://www.habitat.org	Home repair
Military Warriors Support Foundation	https://militarywarriors.org	Mortgage-free homes to veterans with severe injuries
Operation Homefront	http://www.operationhomefront.net	Home repair and modifications for veterans in need
Paralyzed Veterans of America	http://www.pva.org	Broad level of assistance to veterans with spinal cord injuries
Purple Heart Homes	https://www.purplehearthomesusa.org	Help wounded veterans adjust their homes
Semper Fi Fund	https://semperfifund.org	Financial support including for housing needs
The Home Depot Foundation	https://corporate.homedepot.com/community	Grants to organizations that help veterans with homes
Veterans of Foreign Wars	http://www.vfw.org	Assistance to veterans for education, scholarships, activities for youth, filling out forms and claims
Vietnam Veterans of America	http://www.vva.org	Broad range of services

These veterans contributed their service in the following arenas:

- Vietnam (36%)
- Gulf War (1990–present; 28%)
- Peacetime service (23%)
- Korean War (10%)
- World War II (6%)

Note that the first list does not add to 100 percent as some veterans claim to be in "other" or multiple racial/ethnic categories. The second list adds to more than 100 percent because some veterans served in more than one war.

Compared with other Americans, veterans are more likely to have graduated high school (92 percent compared with 88 percent of the national population). Among those aged older than 25 years, they are less likely to have graduated with a four-year college degree (26 percent for veterans compared with 28 percent of the total U.S. population). With a median income of more than $35,000 a year, veterans' annual incomes are about $10,000 higher than that of the average American. It should be recognized that these statistics can vary widely by region, and local data are essential.

California, Texas, and Florida each have more than 1.5 million veterans. This is not surprising because these are highly populated states, ranking 1, 2, and 4 in population, respectively (New York ranks third in population). Looking at the data another way, Alaska, Maine, and Montana have the largest proportion of veterans in their populations, with California and New York having the smallest proportions. Within states, clusters of veterans are primarily found in rural areas of Washington, Oregon, Montana, Texas, Arizona, Alabama, Florida, Michigan, Virginia, and Maine, as well as in small cities. The U.S. Census Bureau reports that more than 20 percent of veterans are located in the following cities,[38,39] all in the south and southwest regions of the nation and all associated with a major military facility:

- Killeen, Texas—Fort Hood
- Clarksville, Tennessee—Fort Campbell
- Jacksonville, North Carolina—Marine Corps Camp Lejeune and Air Station
- Fayetteville, North Carolina—Fort Bragg
- Hampton, Virginia—Langley Air Force Base

The detailed geography of veterans across the United States is interesting. Veterans tend to live near military facilities, in rural areas, and less so in large cities such as New York, New York; Chicago, Illinois; and Los Angeles, California. Yet so many people live in large cities that it is a reality that programs for veterans are needed everywhere.

Government Political Vulnerability

Earlier we noted that investigating political and social processes, especially trigger event(s), is essential for your organization to understand what role it might be called upon to play. When it comes to veterans, political analysis points to vulnerabilities at the federal level. Veterans' organizations have good reasons to voice distress and good reasons to pressure the federal government for change. For example, there was serious anger when the U.S. Congress allowed the 2011 budget sequesters to take effect, slashing programs that veterans and their families depend upon. In 2014, CNN reported "Senate shenanigans capped a winter of discontent for our community in which Washington continually attacked military members, veterans and their families."[40]

Veteran homelessness has become a major political vulnerability. Media reported that 50,000 veterans were homeless, and the Obama administration responded with a program that has been reported to reduce homelessness among veterans by one-third since 2010. VA data show that 11 to 20 percent of post-9/11 veterans and up to 30 percent of Vietnam ones suffer from a form of PTSD, and the result has been a substantial increase in suicides among veterans. Furthermore, many cases of PTSD among veterans are neither diagnosed nor adequately treated.[41] Reports like these imply that the federal government is not sufficiently proactive about veterans' needs. Thus, veterans' organizations have been pressuring the federal government to take action to address these grievances.

Local Level

Stepping back from national politics, some remarkable efforts have been made at the local level, particularly efforts to integrate the needs of veterans into holistic programs. The federal and state governments and the nonprofit and philanthropic organizations listed previously are part of these efforts, but there needs to be creative ways to address homelessness, health care, employment training, and the set of veterans' needs described previously in a coherent fashion.

Homelessness may be the key issue to address at this time. The National Alliance to End Homelessness reports that 91 percent of homeless veterans are male, 76 percent live in a city, and 54 percent have a mental and/or physical disability. Black veterans constitute 39 percent of the homeless veteran population but they only make up 11 percent of the total veteran population. More than 40 percent of homeless veterans are currently aged between 41 and 55 years; thus, the number of homeless veterans aged older than 55 years will substantially increase with time.[42] With strong support from President Obama, the U.S. Department of Housing and Urban Development (HUD) played a central role in trying to eliminate veterans' homelessness. HUD launched a database management system that can be accessed by all interested parties.[43] In cooperation with the Department of Labor, it started a demonstration program focusing on veterans returning from Iraq and Afghanistan, funding programs in nearby proximity to five military installations to provide housing, counseling, and employment counseling[44]:

1. Tampa, Florida—MacDill Air Force Base
2. San Diego, California—Camp Pendleton
3. Killeen, Texas—Fort Hood
4. Watertown, New York—Fort Drum
5. Tacoma, Washington—Joint Base Lewis–McChord

Veterans Village of San Diego

Scores of good local efforts exist in every state. However, not every organization lasts. Based on longevity, creativity, and achievements, we picked Veterans Village of San Diego (VVSD) to illustrate a long-standing model of how to assist veterans. San Diego is a major location for the U.S. military. A year-2011 study asserts that San Diego has the largest concentration of military in the world, including 60 percent of the ships of the U.S. Pacific Fleet and more than 100,000 active-duty Navy and Marine Corps personnel. Using a regional input-output model (see Chapter 9), the analysts estimated that, in fiscal year 2009, direct military spending in the San Diego region led to $30.5 billion in economic impact and approximately 350,000 jobs.[45] The San Diego region includes facilities devoted to training, recruiting, analysis and intelligence, research and development, production, construction, and many other military activities. The following lists some of the well-known military facilities in the San Diego area:

- Camp Pendleton Marine Camp
- Miramar Air Station
- Naval Base Coronado
- Naval Base Point Loma
- Naval Base San Diego
- Naval Medical Center, San Diego
- Recruiting Depot in San Diego

It is not surprising that facilities to assist veterans have been established in the San Diego area. San Diego County is the fifth most populated county in the United States and has the third largest number of veterans. Only Los Angeles County, California, and Maricopa County (Phoenix), Arizona, can boast having more veterans.

The story behind VVSD speaks to the need for coordination among highly motivated and organized individuals with a background in the U.S. military. As reported on the VVSD Web site, the idea originated with five Vietnam War veterans who were dealing with the impacts of war and seeking to do something positive rather than directing their anger at the VA for not helping homeless and distressed veterans. In 1981, the five veterans formed Vietnam Veterans of San Diego, which changed its name to "Veterans Village of San Diego" in 2005. During the past three-plus decades, VVSD built a network of relationships with local and county agencies, the VA, and many others to address homelessness, mental and physical health, and employment challenges.[46–48]

The goals of VVSD are broad. For example, its Web site summarizes what it does as follows:

> VVSD assists homeless veterans who have substance abuse and/or mental health issues, including men and women who have recently returned from Iraq and Afghanistan. The heart of the VVSD's programs is five pillars of success: prevention, intervention, rehabilitation, and aftercare and empowerment services.[48]

The programs use a behavioral model:

> The Veterans Treatment Center (VTC) is a residential program for homeless veterans battling alcoholism, drug addiction and emotional trauma. We believe our program will be the first step toward our veterans' goal of becoming self-sufficient.

The program focuses on helping each veteran to handle their feelings in a healthy way and to identify a new way of living. It is divided into four phases:

1. Assessment and treatment
2. Recovery and treatment
3. Employment development
4. Community reintegration

Each phase involves individual counseling, treatment, and other forms of assistance. Veterans are divided into combat (received fire while in service), co-occurring (serious behavioral health issues and substance use disorders), and chronic relapse (difficulty being sober and has failed treatment efforts) groups.

VVSD's headquarters is on a large tract of land located adjacent to the Pacific Highway. It is 3.2 miles north of the San Diego International Airport (about 7 minutes by auto) and about 5 miles west (7 to 10 minutes by car) from the San Diego Zoo (Figure 7.1). Given the location near an airport and major roads, we might get the impression that the immediate vicinity is unpleasant. EJSCREEN suggests otherwise. The one-mile radius is in the lower 25th percentile in California with regard to the air quality, traffic proximity, waste and industrial facilities, and other environmental contamination metrics. Indeed, as we expanded EJSCREEN out to five miles, the environmental indicators approach the California exposure profiles, especially with regard to traffic proximity. About 12,000 people live within the one-mile radius and 390,000 live within the

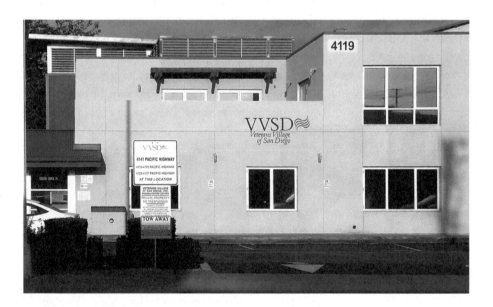

Source: Photo by first author.

Figure 7.1. Veterans Village of San Diego

Table 7.2. Selected Events in Establishing the Veterans Village of San Diego Model

Year	Activity
1981	Vietnam Veterans of San Diego founded
1984	Opened a 44-bed licensed alcohol and drug rehabilitation facility
1988	Founded Stand Down and began to service hundreds of homeless veterans in an 18-bed transitional housing facility
1990–1992	Moved to Pacific Highway location and remodeled a former motel into an 80-bed licensed alcohol and drug rehabilitation center
1995	Established a 44-bed sober living center in Escondido, California
1996	Study completed that praises model treatment program
1997	Opened emergency shelter
1999	Introduced Welcome Home Family Program residential facility for homeless female veterans and their families
2001–2006	Added 80 beds to rehabilitation center (now 165 beds)
2005	Changed its name to "Veterans Village of San Diego" to better reflect its mission
2008	Courtyard added to the rehabilitation center
2009	Further expanded the rehabilitation center with a new intake center and added an employment and training department, medical and administrative facilities
2010	Constructed Veterans On Point Apartments, consisting of 16 three-bedroom, 3-bathroom units
2013	Built affordable housing units, 12 studio apartments with 2 beds each

Source: Based on Veterans Village of San Diego.[46]

five-mile one. The racial/ethnic/socioeconomic mix is not notably different from the region or state as a whole.

VVSD is strong model of how to respond to a moral commitment. In other places, the veteran population may have different priorities. The reader will need to determine what works best for the local environment, and what the best role is for their organization. What this case study shows is that a core of organizers angry at the VA built a model of how to address the problem, how to build a strong organization, gain partners, and slowly but surely add assets by persuading public and private individuals and groups to participate. Table 7.2 shows a chronology of the major changes and accomplishments of the organization.

Case Study: Making Healthy Food Available in Poor Communities

In the veterans' case study, we spent considerable space on national and state, as well as private and public, organizations that have driven efforts to assist veterans. We think providing healthy food is equally challenging but is more dominated by activities at the local level. Hence, this case study pays much more attention to the state and especially local scales. Another way of saying what is presented here is that local planning and health officials are likely to be key if not the major players in providing access to healthy food, whereas they are more likely to play a secondary role in assisting veterans because veterans' groups are highly organized.

Providing healthy food sounds easy enough. It means providing enough food and providing healthy food without disruption. Neither of those activities is easy, however, particularly when the population is poor and lacks transportation. Even in the most economically powerful nations, food supplies have periodically been reduced by droughts and other weather events, wars and political hostilities, and transportation failures that delay food in transit. A great deal has been written by the United Nations, the United States, and other government and nongovernment organizations on what constitutes food security. International organizations estimate that about 900 million people—about 13 percent of the world's population—are food insecure, most living in so-called developing nations.[49,50]

Food insecurity is associated with negative health outcomes. Those with food insecurity self-report poorer health; they are more likely to have poorer mental health and be depressed and to suffer from hypertension; and children with food insecurity are likely to have poor academic records.[51-55] Considerable distress occurred in late 2007, when the following events took place that arguably caused a substantial increase in world food insecurity:

- Economic recession in the United States and elsewhere that changed buying, saving, and other economic decisions
- Increased use of biofuels in the United States, which diverted resources away from growing food
- Increased world oil prices, which increased the cost of growing and transporting food
- Loss of agricultural land to human residential and industrial development
- Increased demand for food in China and India attributable to cumulative increases in population and increasing wealth
- Continuing population growth in developing nations leading to more demand
- Climate events that destroyed food in some countries

The U.S. government pays close attention to food security through the U.S. Department of Agriculture (USDA). The USDA defines food security as "access by all people at all times to enough food for an active, healthy lifestyle."[56] It surveys families every year and produces informative data sets. You can look up food security in your state by going on the USDA Web site. If you do, you will find, not surprisingly, that places with the lowest family incomes almost always have the highest levels of food insecurity. At the state level, Mississippi, Arkansas, Louisiana, Kentucky, and Alabama all fit the expectation for high food insecurity and low income. Texas and Ohio do not. Other factors are in play, however, including unemployment, immigration, race, ethnicity, urban/rural mix, and other factors. Thus, we need to examine these data within states (Table 7.3).

Table 7.3. Rates of Food Insecurity by Selected States, 2014

State	Rank Estimate of Food Insecure (%)	Rank in Family Income
Mississippi	1 (22.0)	50
Arkansas	2 (19.9)	44
Louisiana	3 (17.6)	47
Kentucky	4 (17.5)	46
Texas	5 (17.2)	27
Ohio	6 (16.9)	36
Alabama	7 (16.8)	48
United States, total	(14.3)	NA

Source: Based on U.S. Department of Agriculture.[56]

We chose California for this case study, which is not a state you might expect to be affected by food insecurity because California has historically been one of the most affluent states as measured by household income (ranking third in 2014). It also had a food insecurity rate below the national one (13.5% vs. 14.3%, respectively, in 2014). However, California is the most populous and ethnically/racially diverse state, and it illustrates well the challenges and efforts of both government and private organizations to deal with the complexity of food insecurity.

California's Food Security Dilemma

In June 2012, the University of California Los Angeles (UCLA) Center for Policy Research reported that nearly 4 million California residents were food insecure.[57] They used their annual health interview survey to chart trends in food insecurity across the state with a focus on low-income populations. The number of Californians who could not afford enough food increased from 2.5 million in 2001 to 3.8 million in 2009, a change five times as large as the state's population increase. Notably, 40 percent of California's poor population was food insecure. In 2009, 1.4 million low-income residents of California had very low food security, which means that they had to cut back on the amount of food consumed. Spanish-language residents were at highest risk of food insecurity.[57]

Three counties in California had a total of more than 2 million food insecure people in 2014: Los Angeles, San Diego, and Orange. Among these three, Los Angeles and San Diego counties had lower rates of food insecurity among the poor than the state average. Orange County had the highest food insecurity rate among the poor—52 percent in 2009. The authors attribute some of the increase in food insecurity to the doubling of the unemployment rate between 2007 and 2009, with resultant declines in household incomes.

Employment has since increased and the California economy, like that of the United States, has rebounded.[57] Nevertheless, the need to provide food to the poor continues to be a moral challenge for government. Some local governments in California have developed notable programs that are worthy of more detailed review here because they represent models that might fit other locations in the United States.

We begin by noting that Orange County ranks sixth out of 58 counties in family income in California. Yet, 24 percent of the population is poor, and, overall, 11 percent of the population is defined as food insecure. Garcia-Silva and colleagues[58] reported on Orange County's efforts, with the County Public Health Officer and the Director of the County Food Bank, starting the Waste Not OC Coalition (WNOC). The organization set out three objectives:

1. Identify food-insecure individuals.
2. Educate the population about food donations.
3. Connect food-insecure individuals to food sources.

To build a network tying needy people together with food, WNOC partnered with a not-for-profit that picks up food from restaurants, other businesses, and hospitals, and delivers it to food pantries. Garcia-Silva and colleagues[58] also noted that the health department plays a key role through its inspectors who visit food facilities two to three times a year. The results of these efforts include the following:

- Twenty-five food pantries have signed on as recipients and the number continues to increase.
- A new supermarket joined the group and promised food donations, as have some schools and other private donors.
- The local children's hospital has screened patients for food insecurity and provided some with food and information about the food pantries.
- The group is developing an education module to make sure that food pantries understand how the food can be kept fresh.

At the time we wrote this chapter, there was apparently some local resistance to this program, but the authors note that WNOC has already had an impact in providing needed food. This is a relatively new program, and its claims are modest. However, it is the kind of program that can be implemented in many locations across the United States without a massive infusion of resources. The social network required to start such a program is small and replicable in other places. The key to success is how they recruit contributors and screen potential clients.

Community Health Councils of Los Angeles

Community Health Councils (CHC) is a nonprofit community health promotion and policy organization in Los Angeles. It was organized in 1992[59] after the major civil unrest in that city following the acquittal of the officers in the Rodney King case. CHC is a model of how to galvanize efforts around human health issues in large, poor communities. Gabriel Stover, former director of research and evaluation at CHC, reports that local physicians and key neighborhood leaders focused on the lack of health care services in this community of more than 700,000 residents (G. Stover, telephone communication, August 21, 2016). A network of health-oriented members gathered around this core group, first at the neighborhood level and later to be joined by the health department, planning department, and the mayor's office. Lark Galloway-Gilliam, the executive director, is credited as the key leader who knew how to organize and expand the network and to secure external support.[60] The Web site states that

> CHC's mission is to promote social justice and achieve equity in communities and environmental resources to improve the health of underserved populations.[59]

CHC's organizational approach is to build coalitions and mobilize supporters, including community leaders, consumer advocates, faith-based leaders, and practitioners from the health care, social service, and education communities. Eight specific focal points are listed on its Web site[59]:

- Health reform
- Public reporting on the quality of health care
- Preserving the health care safety net
- Tobacco and air quality control
- Regulation of urban oil drilling
- Expanded walking, biking, and public transportation options
- Increased park and open spaces
- A diversity of resources for fresh, wholesome food

This large agenda leads CHC to conduct community-based research, offer community-based policy recommendations, disseminate information, offer educational programs, and build a large network from among public and private organizations. CHC's funders include 15 private and public organizations, including the Annenberg Foundation and the Robert Wood Johnson Foundation.

One of the many organizational strengths of the CHC is its relationship with UCLA. This has led to a published portfolio of 25 reports that are Web-accessible. Seven of these reports are primarily about food and nutrition. Table 7.4 summarizes the two more recent reports.

The context for the studies in Table 7.4 is the marked rise in childhood obesity and its implications for heart disease and diabetes. The areas targeted for this work have among the highest or the highest rates of morbidity and mortality for these diseases in Los Angeles and California as a whole. Children in South Los Angeles consume more fast food and sugar-sweetened beverages and less fruits and vegetables than other children

Table 7.4. Community Health Councils Health Impact Assessments Regarding Food Quality in South Los Angeles

Study	Methods and Recommendations
Street Vendor Legalization and Student Nutrition in South Los Angeles Health Impact Assessment, 2015[61]	*Methods:* Use HIA to compare the presence of street vendors and types of food consumed near public schools with and without regulations regarding street vendor presence and practices. *Findings:* Street vendor regulations are not consistently enforced and are ineffective. *Recommendations:* More enforcement combined with encouragement of healthy food not only among street vendors but also in nearby food outlets are both essential.
South Los Angeles Fast Food Health Impact Assessment, 2013[62]	*Methods:* Use HIA to better understand proposed land use changes in regard to fast food restaurants. *Findings:* Existing regulations have slowed spread of fast food restaurants but not stopped their expansion. *Recommendations:* End loopholes that have allowed expansion and tighten or maintain current density of fast food restaurant requirements; exempt "healthy" restaurants from regulations; incorporate HIAs in planning process.

Source: Based on Baird (2015)[61]; Morrison (2013).[63]
Note: HIA = health impact assessment.

and have the highest obesity in Los Angeles County.[63] Both HIAs were completed in response to legislative proposals regarding the location of fast food outlets and street vendors in Los Angeles.

Figure 7.2 is the logic tree for the street vendor HIA study. Table 7.5 compares the options for restricting fast food restaurants examined in the fast food HIA.

EJSCREEN provides a sense of the relative burden of environmental challenges for those living in South Los Angeles. We placed a pin at the center of the South Los Angeles district and drew a two-mile radius around the pin in order to include Southeast Los Angeles and the West Adams areas, both of which are relatively poor. The population density of the area is 8,200 per square mile; 98 percent of the residents are minorities, nearly all Hispanic and/or black. The per capita income of the area is about half of that for Los Angeles County as a whole. These are unenviable environmental metrics. Compared with the State of California, this two-mile-radius area was in the 90th to 98th percentile with regard to exposures to PM 2.5 and lead paint, as well as proximity to traffic, NPL sites, waste management, and water discharge areas. Ozone, a regional contaminant, was at about the 80th percentile for California. In short, this environmentally stressed area is a key part of CHC's agenda.

From the start of the CHC's program, we see an evolution of thinking and analysis as follows:

- Understand literature linking poor nutrition to disease outcomes in adults and children.

- Investigate the number and density of fast food, grocery, mom-and-pop food stores, and street vendors, as well as determine sources of high-quality food.
- Understand how government can reduce access to less nutritious foods through zoning, especially use of density restrictions for fast-food stores.
- Learn how to use incentives and marketing to attract high-quality grocery stores, sit-down restaurants, farmer's markets, local gardens, and other sources of higher quality food.
- Provide educational programs to persuade the community to support the higher quality food.
- Offer evidence-based research that connects nutritional food policy to public policy options.

Detailed population analyses and surveys were part of this program; environmental and social justice research is part of the core of this group's work. HIAs were used in these two reports, and CHC recommends the use of HIAs in its work. In other words, CHC has used every tool reviewed in this chapter and those in Chapter 5 with one exception. It did not use EJSCREEN, most probably because the tool was not available until after CHC's most recent food-related report was published. The list of interconnected but clear objectives published by CHC shows the organization's understanding of the importance of building networks and allies to achieve its goals.

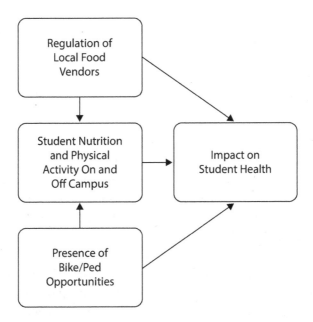

Source: Based on Baird (2015).[61]

Figure 7.2. Health Impact Assessment Logic Model for Street Vendor Study

Table 7.5. Review of Options for Limiting Fast Food Restaurants in Los Angeles

Topic	Current General Plan Amendment	Proposed West Adams Plan Policies
Density limitations for freestanding fast food restaurants	Half-mile distance requirement for freestanding fast food restaurants with exemption for Council District 10 North of 10 Freeway	Half-mile distance requirement for freestanding fast food restaurants with exemption for entire Council District 10 portion of West Adams except in TODs
Density limitations for freestanding fast food restaurants in TODs	No special designation of TOD areas	Quarter-mile density boundary and designated TOD areas
Density limitations for freestanding fast food restaurants near schools	No special designation of school areas	Restriction of fast food restaurant development adjacent to or near schools in designated areas
Costs to developer for receiving an exemption	$23,000 exemption filing fee	Approximately $17,000 exemption filing fee
Pedestrian corridor design standards for freestanding fast food	No special designation of pedestrian corridors	30-foot setback in pedestrian corridors
Density limitations for drive-through fast food restaurants	750-foot density boundary for drive-through restaurants in Hyde Park and Leimert Park	750-foot density boundary for drive-through restaurants in Hyde Park and Leimert Park
Density limitations for freestanding fast food restaurants	No special designation for freestanding fast food restaurants	Half-mile density boundary for freestanding fast food restaurants (except in Council District 10)
Density limitations for freestanding fast food restaurants in TODs	No special designation of TOD areas	Quarter-mile density boundary in designated TOD areas

Source: Based on Morrison (2013).[62]
Note: TOD = transit-oriented development.

Final Thoughts

Responding to legal obligations and moral commitments can badly divide a community or it can make it much stronger. Public health and planning officials, whether by choice or not, become key players in developing and implementing responses. They must understand the social and political origins of the programs to which they are responding to avoid making serious errors that will undermine their efforts. They should jointly set out clear goals with measurable objectives with the groups with which they will interact. Those goals should make sense for their community and be based on political reality— the likely reaction of political leadership to recommended solutions. Social network analysis, EJSCREEN, and assessment of political and social processes will help those addressing challenges to achieve the needed level of understanding. Public outreach tools, analysis and mapping of census and other data, and perhaps collaborative processes and HIA will be valuable.

References

1. Seley JE. *The Politics of Public-Facility Planning.* Lexington, MA: Lexington Books; 1983.

2. De Nooy W, Mrvar A, Batagelj V. *Exploratory Social Network Analysis With Pajek.* 2nd ed. New York, NY: Cambridge University Press; 2011.

3. Mislove A, Marcon M, Gummadi K, Druschel P, Bhatacharjee B. Measurement and analysis of online social networks. In: *IMC'07, October 24–26.* San Diego, CA; 2007.

4. Fowler JH, Christakis NA. Dynamic spread of happiness in a large social network: longitudinal analysis over 20 years in the Framingham Heart Study. *BMJ.* 2008;337(7531):a2338.

5. Pearson M. Social network analysis: an overview. Employment Research Institute, Edinburgh Napier University. 2013. Available at: http://www.napier.ac.uk/~/media/worktribe/output-187063/socialnetworkanalysisreviewdraftmppdf.ashx. Accessed March 10, 2017.

6. Ennett ST, Bailey SL, Federman EB. Social network characteristics associated with risky behaviors among runaway and homeless youth. *J Health Soc Behav.* 1999;40(1):63.

7. Christakis NA, Fowler JH. The spread of obesity in a large social network over 32 years. *N Engl J Med.* 2007;357(4):370–379.

8. Cohen-Cole E, Fletcher JM. Is obesity contagious? Social networks vs. environmental factors in the obesity epidemic. *J Health Econ.* 2008;27(5):1382–1387.

9. Friedman M. Posttraumatic stress disorder among military returnees from Afghanistan and Iraq. *Am J Psychiatry.* 2006;16(4):586–593.

10. Pietrzak R, Johnson D, Goldstein M. Psychosocial buffers of traumatic stress, depressive symptoms, and psychosocial difficulties in veterans of Operations Enduring Freedom and Iraqi Freedom: the role. *J Affect.* 2010;129(1):188–192.

11. Boscarino J. Post-traumatic stress and associated disorders among Vietnam veterans: the significance of combat exposure and social support. *J Trauma Stress.* 1995;8:317–226.

12. Mares A, Kasprow W, Rosenheck R. Outcomes of supported housing for homeless veterans with psychiatric and substance abuse problems. *Ment Heal Serv.* 2004;6(4):199–211.

13. Whatmore S, Thorne L. Nourishing networks: alternative geographies of food. In: Goodman D, Watts M, eds. *Globalizing Food: Agrarian Questions and Global Restructuring.* London, England: Routledge; 1997:287–304.

14. Hamelin A-M, Habicht J-P, Beaudry M. Symposium: Advances in Measuring Food Insecurity and Hunger in the US Food insecurity: consequences for the household and broader social implications 1. *J Nutr.* 1999;129:525–528.

15. Ahluwalia IB, Dodds JM, Baligh M. Social support and coping behaviors of low-income families experiencing food insufficiency in North Carolina. *Health Educ Behav.* 1998;25(5):599–612.

16. Dhokarh R, Himmelgreen DA, Peng Y-K, Segura-Pérez S, Hromi-Fiedler A, Pérez-Escamilla R. Food insecurity is associated with acculturation and social networks in Puerto Rican households. *J Nutr Educ Behav*. 2011;43(4):288–294.

17. Campbell MC. Building a common table: the role for planning in community food systems. *J Plan Educ Res*. 2004;23(4):341–355.

18. US Environmental Protection Agency. Environmental justice. Available at: https://www.epa.gov/environmentaljustice. Accessed August 21, 2016.

19. US Environmental Protection Agency. EJSCREEN: Environmental Justice Screening and Mapping Tool. Available at: https://www.epa.gov/ejscreen. Accessed August 21, 2016.

20. Hanna-Attisha M, LaChance J. Elevated blood lead levels in children associated with the Flint drinking water crisis: a spatial analysis of risk and public health response. *Am J Public Health*. 2016;106(2):283–290.

21. McAdam D, Tarrow S, Tilly C. *Dynamics of Contention*. New York, NY: Cambridge University Press; 2001.

22. McAdam D. *Political Process and the Development of Black Insurgency, 1930–1970*. 2nd ed. Chicago, IL: University of Chicago Press; 1982.

23. Morris AD. *The Origins of the Civil Rights Movement: Black Communities Organizing for Change*. New York, NY: Free Press; 1984.

24. Jonas G. *Freedom's Sword: The NAACP and the Struggle Against Racism in America, 1909–1969*. New York, NY: Routledge; 2005.

25. Weiss NJ. *The National Urban League, 1910–1940*. New York, NY: Oxford University Press; 1974.

26. Ball H. *A Defiant Life: Thurgood Marshall and the Persistence of Racism in America*. New York, NY: Crown Publishers; 1998.

27. Kotz N. *Judgment Days: Lyndon Baines Johnson, Martin Luther King Jr., and the Laws That Changed America*. Boston, MA: Houghton Mifflin; 2005.

28. Karabell Z, Rosenberg J. *Kennedy, Johnson, and the Quest for Justice: The Civil Rights Tapes*. New York, NY: W.W. Norton & Company; 2003.

29. McWhorter D. *Carry Me Home: Birmingham, Alabama: The Climactic Battle of the Civil Rights Revolution*. New York, NY: Simon & Schuster; 2001.

30. Dudziak ML. *Cold War Civil Rights: Race and the Image of American Democracy (Politics and Society in Modern America)*. Princeton, NJ: Princeton University Press; 2011.

31. National Advisory Commission on Civil Disorders. Report of the National Advisory Commission on Civil Rights. 1967. Available at: http://www.eisenhowerfoundation.org/docs/kerner.pdf. Accessed August 21, 2016.

32. US Department of Veterans Affairs. Housing assistance—homeless veterans. Available at: http://www.va.gov/homeless/housing.asp. Accessed March 9, 2017.

33. US Interagency Council on Homelessness. Veterans and families focus of April 2015 Council Meeting. 2015. Available at: https://www.usich.gov. Accessed March 9, 2017.

34. US Department of Housing and Urban Development. Veterans Affairs Supportive Housing. Available at: http://portal.hud.gov/hudportal/HUD?src=/program_offices/public_indian_housing/programs/hcv/vash. Accessed March 9, 2017.

35. US Department of Defense Office of Warrior Care Policy. National Resource Directory. Available at: http://warriorcare.dodlive.mil/nrd. Accessed March 9, 2017.

36. The White House. Joining forces. 2014. Available at: https://www.whitehouse.gov/joiningforces. Accessed March 9, 2017.

37. New Jersey Department of Military and Veterans Affairs. New Jersey Veterans' Benefits Guide. 2014. Available at: http://www.nj.gov/military/veterans/njguide/njvet.pdf. Accessed August 21, 2016.

38. US Census Bureau. A snapshot of our nation's veterans. 2012. Available at: https://www.census.gov/content/dam/Census/library/visualizations/2012/comm/veterans.pdf. Accessed August 21, 2016.

39. Veterans in the United States. Where soldiers come from. PBS. November 10, 2011. Available at: http://www.pbs.org/pov/wheresoldierscomefrom/photo-gallery-map-veterans-usa/2. Accessed March 9, 2017.

40. Rieckhoff P. Congress lets down military families and vets. CNN. March 4, 2014. Available at: http://www.cnn.com/2014/03/04/opinion/rieckhoff-congress-military-vets. Accessed March 9, 2017.

41. Quil L. The US declared war on veteran homelessness—and it actually could win. National Public Radio. August 4, 2015. Accessed March 9, 2017.

42. National Alliance to End Homelessness. FAQs 2017. Available at: http://www.endhomelessness.org/?library/entry/fact-sheeet-veteran-homeless. Accessed March 9, 2017.

43. US Department of Housing and Urban Development. Tackling veteran homelessness with HUDStat. Evidence matters. 2012. Available at: https://www.huduser.gov/portal/periodicals/em/summer12/highlight1.html. Accessed March 9, 2017.

44. US Department of Housing and Urban Development. VHPD: Veterans Homelessness Prevention Demonstration Program—HUD exchange. 2015. Available at: https://www.hudexchange.info/programs/vhpd. Accessed March 9, 2017.

45. San Diego Military Advisory Council. San Diego Military Economic Impact Study. 2011. Available at: https://www.sdmac.org/ImpactStudy.htm. Accessed March 9, 2017.

46. Veterans Village of San Diego. VVSD history. 2010. Available at: http://www.vvsd.net/history.htm. Accessed March 9, 2017.

47. Veterans Village of San Diego. "Leave no one behind." 2010. Available at: http://vvsd.net. Accessed March 9. 2017.

48. Veterans Village of San Diego. Veterans Treatment Center. 2010. Available at: http://www. vvsd.net/vtc.htm. Accessed March 9, 2017.

49. Food and Agriculture Organization of the United Nations. The state of food insecurity in the world. 2015. Available at: http://www.fao.org/hunger/en. Accessed March 9, 2017.

50. World Hunger Education Service. 2016 world hunger and poverty facts and statistics. Available at: http://www.worldhunger.org/2015-world-hunger-and-poverty-facts-and-statistics. Accessed March 9, 2017.

51. Jyoti DF, Frongillo EA, Jones SJ. Food insecurity affects school children's academic performance, weight gain, and social skills. *J Nutr*. 2005;135(12):2831–2839.

52. Larson NI, Story MT. Food insecurity and weight status among US children and families: a review of the literature. *Am J Prev Med*. 2011;40(2):166–173.

53. Tarasuk VS. Household food insecurity with hunger is associated with women's food intakes, health and household circumstances. *J Nutr*. 2001;131(10):2670–2676.

54. Whitaker RC, Phillips SM, Orzol SM. Food insecurity and the risks of depression and anxiety in mothers and behavior problems in their preschool-aged children. *Pediatrics*. 2006;118(3): e859–e868.

55. Seligman HK, Laraia BA, Kushel MB. Food insecurity is associated with chronic disease among low-income NHANES participants. *J Nutr*. 2010;140(2):304–310.

56. US Department of Agriculture, Economic Research Service. Food security in the US 2014. Available at: http://www.ers.usda.gov/topics/food-nutrition-assistance/food-security-in-the-us.aspx. Accessed August 21, 2016.

57. Chaparro MP, Langellier B, Birnbach K, Sharp K, Harrison G. Nearly four million Californians are food insecure. UCLA Health Policy Brief. 2012. Available at: https://escholarship. org/uc/item/5407m7mh. Accessed August 21, 2016.

58. Garcia-Silva B, Handler E, Wolfe J. A public–private partnership to mitigate food insecurity and food waste in Orange County, California. *Am J Public Health*. 2017;107(1):105.

59. Community Health Councils. About CHC. Available at: http://chc-inc.org/about-chc-1. Accessed March 9, 2017.

60. California Pan-Ethnic Health Network. Voices for health equity. Available at: http://cpehn. org/blog/lags/community-health-councils-inc. Accessed May 5, 2016.

61. Baird R. *Street Vendor Legalization and Student Nutrition in South Los Angeles: Health Impact Assessment*. Los Angeles, CA: Community Health Councils; 2015.

62. Morrison B. *South LA Fast Food Health Impact Assessment*. Los Angeles, CA: Community Health Councils; 2013.

63. Wolstein J, Babey SH, Diamant AL. *Obesity in California*. Los Angeles, CA: UCLA Center for Health Policy Research; 2015.

8

REDEVELOPING AN EYESORE: HOW SAFE IS SAFE ENOUGH?

This chapter introduces three tools that may be used by decision-makers when dealing with major redevelopment projects that carry the potential for serious human health and safety risks. The redevelopment project may need all or some of the following actions: investigation of the site for human health and safety risks, demolition, excavation, pump and treat to reduce concentration of contaminants in groundwater, remediation, or security barriers to prevent ingress of humans or egress of contaminants. In some cases it may require new construction with a plan for reuse and/or long-term stewardship. Major redevelopment projects are among the most challenging for public health and planning officials insofar as they require close interaction throughout the decision-making and implementation stages. When stewardship is appropriate, it requires a long-term commitment to monitor engineered systems and institutional controls. This is demonstrated through a case study of a sustainably protective waste management system at the Fernald Preserve, Ohio, site, a Department of Energy (DOE) former uranium processing facility. The tools covered in this chapter include the following:

- Collaborative problem solving
- Planning and design charrettes
- Risk analysis: risk assessment and management

Collaborative Problem Solving

Before making a redevelopment decision that will impact a large number of people, it is prudent to obtain information about public preferences, perceptions, and values. This might be done by conducting surveys face to face, through the mail, on the Web, or over the phone. Data collected via surveys are best obtained through a random process (i.e., one in which every eligible person has a chance to be selected) so that the results approximate the views of the actual population potentially impacted. Another method for gathering data about public preferences on redevelopment is to use focus groups. Typically, a group of six to eight people representing a specific part of the community (e.g., senior citizens, residents of the East Ward) is guided through a discussion to ascertain their views. Someone takes notes, usually on large pads sitting on easels or on white boards, and uses the notes to represent the views of the larger population. Focus groups and surveys are often used in tandem. They can produce valuable data about preferences for redevelopment options. For example, given that a community has restricted financial resources, does the group think those resources should be used to redevelop a shopping mall, or should they be used to demolish an old factory and replace it with a new school?

A third way to assess public preferences about redevelopment is to hold public meetings; however, this normally means one-way dissemination of information by the meeting organizers and allows for limited responses by attendees. Public meetings are typically conducted because they are legally required. Someone that is part of the team that organized the meeting should be taking notes, using a tape recorder or on a white board or other surface for a postmeeting debriefing. There may be follow-up meetings or not depending upon legal mandates and budgets. Although public meetings are appropriate to introduce an issue, they are often ineffective at getting to the heart of what people want and are willing to live with. Public meetings are often dominated by speakers who do not know when to stop talking and/or showing slides and by outspoken individuals trying to score points, often for media consumption.

Focus groups and surveys are far better ways of learning about the population's perceptions, preferences, and values on big issues. Unfortunately, when many options for redevelopment are possible, these tools become less effective. When decision-makers want to ascertain what people really want for a large redevelopment project that presents many options, the answer may lie in a collaborative problem-solving process.

When a group of people work together to choose from a variety of options until they arrive at a consensus, they are said to be engaged in collaborative decision-making.[1-6] In other words, the decision is attributable to a group working together rather than to only one or a few people. The decision, then, should be reflective of the group's collective preferences, perceptions, and values. In a democratic society, collaborative processes are desirable because they include many perspectives and should reduce polarization about decisions. A caution, however, is that, although the authors believe in and have participated in collaborative processes, the process does not guarantee better results as measured by short- or long-term indicators of human health and safety. A collaborative process may produce results that are heavily weighted to create jobs or to increase tax revenues and other outcomes rather than to prioritize health and safety measures. Collaborative processes demand time, as well as human and capital resources that may not be available.

Collaborative processes differ from focus groups, surveys, and public meetings for learning about public preferences. A group consensus-building process typically consists of 8 to 30 people. The group members bring different information, values, perceptions, and preferences with them. A group leader, often a professional facilitator, provides all of the members of the group with the same information, tries to reduce their differences, and builds trust. In the end, the group tries to reach a unanimous agreement, but sometimes that is not possible. Hence, they must decide if they will agree on majority rule. If they will not and if everyone has to agree, then they must negotiate until there is a consensus that all members can live with, even if some are not happy with the outcome.

Some technical tools may be used when groups are relatively large and meetings are difficult to arrange. One of these is the Delphi Method, an analytical process tool used to arrive at a consensus decision.[7] The essence of the method is to identify a group and to periodically provide feedback to its members about what each thinks about given issues. Time is then allowed for members of the group to revise their views after which the process of feedback begins again until consensus is reached. There is no universally accepted protocol for who should lead the communications provided to the participants, or what types of communication mechanisms should be used. In the absence of enough meetings to establish trust among the participants, there is a danger that the leader of the group may overplay his/her role, resulting in some members of the group dropping out. Although the loss of disenchanted members of the group may make other members of the group happy, it may also lead to a faulty consensus decision that will not be widely accepted by the larger population. In our experience, the Delphi Method works best when the group has a membership with very diverse backgrounds and experiences and, most importantly, it is otherwise difficult for group members to meet face-to-face and discuss their views.

Other collaborative process tools allow participants to vote on options, with the option garnering the highest amount of support being selected. One variant of consensus voting is a formal process called "dot voting." Dot voting uses an idea rating sheet where the pollster, group leader, or facilitator places an option (statement) at the top of the voting form and then members of the voting group add their dot indicating how well they agree with the option as presented.[8] Idea rating sheets yield a spectrum of agreement on an option rather than a simple up or down vote. The idea-rating sheets allow the voters to provide comments, giving important feedback to the facilitator who can then recraft the statement and repeat the dot voting process until a consensus is achieved.

All collaborative processes have limitations. It is important that they focus on information that everyone has access to, which ideally should allow members to narrow down their differences. However, some participants may be unable or unwilling to bargain with regard to options that challenge their values. This means that sometimes it will be impossible for groups to reach common ground when an ideological stance is articulated and held throughout the process. When underlying issues, typically centering on values and experiences, are neglected, they will likely undermine the decision-making process and/or its implementation.

Assume that a redevelopment objective is so important to everyone (public health, planning, and other community stakeholders) that a consensus outcome will be agreed upon, or at least tolerated, by all. Before beginning the process, the organizers need to define "success." Does success mean that everyone agrees with all aspects of the final decision, or will agreement by the majority be sufficient in all or some parts of the process? Once success is defined, there is a relatively standard stepwise progression for the collaborative problem-solving process (Table 8.1).

After the collaborative decision-making process is completed and the option selected has begun to be implemented, implementation must be monitored. Monitoring is important as it may be difficult to fully implement every aspect of a complex decision, and transparency is essential to maintain public trust. Implementation may not happen smoothly for a variety of reasons: a technology that was supposed to work perhaps did not; the budget for implementation may have been drastically cut; or there may be actual efforts to undermine the decision made by consensus. The consensus group may need to be satisfied with outcomes that are less than what was agreed upon or with a time frame that makes success much longer to achieve. Problems with implementation

Table 8.1. Steps in the Collaborative Problem-Solving Process

1. Identify the issue(s) with sufficient precision that the facilitator and group feel that a consensus-building approach will work and that methods such as a town meeting, focus groups, and surveys are not going to be used.

2. Identify parties to participate (people who represent a range of ideas, especially those from groups that if not included could sabotage the group's work).

3. Determine where to meet, someone to monitor/facilitate the process, and the financial resources to pay for the process. Lack of financial backing can be a show stopper and multiple facilitated sessions with reporting back can be expensive. Foundations or the federal/state government may not pay for collaborative decision-making without assurance that the results mirror their preference for a particular outcome.

4. Organize the process to meet the needs of the participants, to determine if participants are able to work together. Organization normally takes one of three paths: start with the relatively easy issues first, then go to the harder ones; vice versa; or divide the issues into categories and create committees to make initial recommendations for those issues that are the most problematic.

5. Define the issues in ways that are sensitive to the range of perceptions, values, and likely initial preferences in the group. For example, a proposed airport will be seen by some as more jobs, taxes, and income. To others, it will be viewed as a locally unwanted land use that will defile the area (see Denver International Airport case study in Chapter 9). Issues need to be defined in ways that will not break up the group process.

6. Define enough plausible options so that all participants feel that their ideas are being considered. After some discussion among the full group or subgroups, members should discuss tradeoffs among options that will bring them closer to a consensus. There are bound to be some factual disagreements, and it is important that group members are involved in determining how these are going to be resolved.

7. Choose a decision and resolve differences among the parties. If this is a near consensus, then press to resolve differences, which is easier to say than to do.

8. Formally choose an option. This may be difficult because if a participant is representing a larger group, s/he may have a difficult time persuading colleagues to sign on.

9. Implement the choice. This can be the most difficult step as it means making sure that what was agreed upon is followed, that there are sufficient resources to allow implementation, and that someone has not changed the chosen option.

may wreak havoc with the credibility of the locally responsible group, lead to legal challenges, and force a renegotiation when everyone thought an issue was settled.

Planning and Design Charrettes

Whenever an opportunity exists to redevelop an existing site and/or build on a new one, and when time, resources, and expertise are available, charrettes should be considered.[9] Technically, a charrette is one or more sessions during which experts present long-range plans and specific designs and the community or its representatives respond to the expert presentation. In our experience, when a charrette contributes to a successful collaboration, parties almost always feel very positive about the outcomes.

Planning charrettes consider variations in use, location, density, scope, and overall cost. Assume that a set of industrial properties located on 100 acres along a major river has been or will soon be abandoned. Some of the properties are contaminated, others are not, and still others are partly occupied and may or may not be contaminated. A planning charrette exercise may posit, for instance, three future uses for this soon-to-be-available 100-acre site:

1. A wholesaling–redistribution center for goods to be brought in by rail and redistributed by rail and highway
2. A sports complex for the entire region, including trying to lure a minor league baseball franchise to a new stadium, and adding additional retail shops to the area
3. Open space for the region, including public playing fields

These very different options have major implications for the community's economy and social network, as well as for public health and the local environment. A local elected official could turn the process over to a developer and/or expert for some ideas. But developers and experts are not necessarily knowledgeable about the preferences of the local community and should not presume to know the desires of the entire region. It is likely that some communities would want a sports complex–retailing package, some might prefer the open space, and others the wholesaling–redistribution idea. Is it smart for local officials to turn the decision about developing the area over to an outside expert/developer? Should there be a process that obtains local input, or should a developer/expert be charged with setting up a process to obtain local input on the three ideas?

When public input is sought, experts should prepare a planning charrette and present it to a representative group relying on sketches, drawings, and illustrations of what the area might look like and how it will relate to the surrounding area. The audience size for this type of charrette is typically 15 to 30 participants. Given this relatively small audience, participants should be prepared to respond with constructive suggestions or at least helpful criticisms. The organizer may use the first meeting to refine their ideas and come back at least one more time or until a consensus emerges about preferences that can be expressed as possible projects with realistic budgets. At some point, the process shifts from a planning charrette to a design one, requiring architects, planners, and others to prepare drawings or a physical model of what the area might look like. The most interesting of these is when designers build a physical or computer model and the group is able to move the pieces around the site and engage in a conversation about options.

The charrette is intended to develop a vision for an area based on stakeholder and expert interactions. During the charrette, experts gather information about group preferences and the reasons for those preferences. On the other hand, charrettes are difficult to organize, especially because facilities must accommodate different kinds of displays and provide participants opportunities for moving objects. These exercises can be very intense, with participants demonstrating their reactions to designs, sometimes with less-than-flattering language and physical gestures. A great deal of emotion, both positive and negative, may be displayed during charrettes. Creating a vision for an area based on stakeholder and expert interactions means that group members learn more about each other and the experts during the charrette process, which is important because it builds trust. Some of the most transparent exchanges of information and ideas that we have witnessed take place during charrettes. The strengths and weaknesses of the charrette process are summarized in Table 8.2.

Figure 8.1 summarizes the decision-making processes that impact how officials might obtain and present information to the public. Note that collaborative decision-making stands out because of its greater complexity and demand for time and resources. In cases in which public health and planning practitioners are involved, the process can be

Table 8.2. Strengths and Weaknesses of Planning and Design Charrettes

Strengths	Weaknesses
• Participants can create a plan and design that is more agreeable to the population and more economical to the developers than could have been expected. • Charrettes can establish positive relationships that continue beyond the life of the project.	• Charrettes involve high costs of time, resource needs, and expertise. • Charrettes are high intensity, beyond the ability of some participants to cope. • The process may be dominated by a few participants for whom the process is more suitable. • There may be lack of participation by some of the most knowledgeable participants because of other commitments and unwillingness to express their views in public. • There may be failure to reach a consensus at either the planning or design stages, despite a major investment of time and resources.

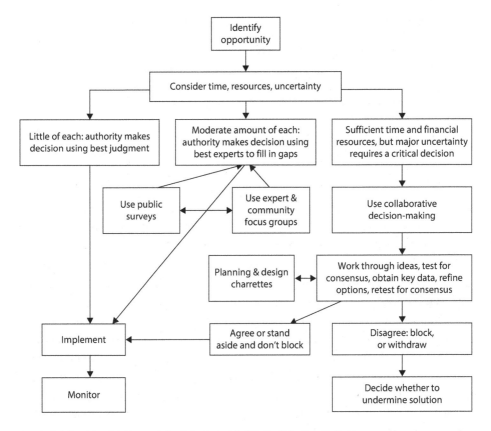

Figure 8.1. Decision-Making and the Selection of Public Participation Option

facilitated by the use of planning and design charrettes, leading to a truly win–win outcome. But to succeed, the process must be supported by expertise and resources, have sufficient time to allow it to flourish, and, most of all, must be joined by devoted participants willing to give their time and energy to the process.

Risk Analysis: Risk Assessment and Risk Management

Those who assess risk and those charged with managing it have distinct challenges. Risk assessors pose and attempt to answer three questions related to the likelihood of a hazard event and its aftermath[10]:

1. What can go wrong?
2. What are the chances that something with serious consequences will go wrong?
3. What are the consequences if something does go wrong?

By contrast, risk managers pose and attempt to answer three different questions:

1. How can consequences be prevented or reduced?
2. How can recovery be enhanced (improve resilience) if the event occurs?
3. How can key local officials, expert staff, and the public organize and be informed to reduce risk and concern and increase trust and confidence?

This chapter assumes that redevelopment poses risks. The first three questions are relatively simple assessment questions, but they do not imply simple answers. When hazards from redevelopment are dangerous and could cause cascading effects that spread across the landscape, when uncertainty is high, and when the consequences could be quite destructive to a large population, then very detailed risk assessments will be required. Luckily, few redevelopment projects pose such high risks and less demanding analyses are usually required, at least during preliminary stages.

This section re-introduces a generic checklist presented in Chapter 5, then adds a semiquantitative approach that is part checklist and part risk assessment. Lastly, it discusses a full-blown risk assessment and risk management process applied to the complex cleanup of a former nuclear weapons site.

Checklists were first discussed and illustrated in Chapter 5. Table 5.1 is a good one to use in this case and in many circumstances in which a new facility is being built, or an existing facility is being remediated and rebuilt. These questions start with a simple probe, and if the answer to that question is "yes," then further investigations are warranted.[11,12]

The checklist questions in Chapter 5 (Table 5.1) can be used in a public or town meeting and are recommended as part of a consensus-building process focusing on a proposed development or redevelopment opportunity in an area. The questions allow participants to cover a set of common human health issues, to comment on them, and to inform experts about other risks that they are concerned about, which then can be added to the checklist. Although public concerns are not necessarily the risks that are most threatening to human health and safety, they nevertheless serve as an icebreaker to get people to talk about the risk-related issues important to them. In other words, a checklist represents a tool that can engage community members in a discussion about their concerns about risk-related issues in a proposed project.

The checklist tool in Table 5.1 can engage community members in a discussion about their concerns about a proposed project. But it is generic—that is, it is meant to begin discussion and identify areas of concern so that nothing important to stakeholders is missed. Experts have developed a set of semiquantitative checklist models that assess risks across many hazardous waste sites in a way that are both transparent and replicable (e.g., they can be readily shared with the public). The models can be applied to assessing human health and safety at waste management sites, as well as at old brownfield and grayfield sites where there is potential exposure to contaminants. This approach takes the user from the forest into the trees. These tools are particularly important when there are hundreds, even thousands, of sites, and priorities must be set to determine where limited

Table 8.3. Process–Model Checklist for Hazardous Waste Sites

1. Determine if the site is hazardous.	✓ Analyze the toxicity of the five most hazardous substances on the site.
	✓ Determine the quantity of these substances on the site.
	✓ Indicate how persistent they are in the environment.
	✓ Measure their concentrations on the site.
	✓ Indicate how well they are contained on the site.
	✓ Indicate the potential for direct public access to the site.
2. Identify exposure pathways from the hazardous substances on the site.	✓ Air exposure.
	✓ Groundwater exposure.
	✓ Surface water exposure.
	✓ Exposure to soil deposited on the site or removed to an off-site location.
	✓ Evidence that the substances have entered the food chain.
3. Look for evidence of human exposure.	✓ Direct knowledge of a potentially exposed population.
	✓ Evidence for human exposure/absorption.
	✓ Evidence found through sampling.
4. Examine health effects.	✓ Reports and allegations of exposure.
	✓ Clinical or epidemiological studies.
	✓ Expected current or acute or short-term effects.
	✓ Expected chronic effects.
	✓ Severity of the expected effects.

Source: Based on Marsh and Day (1991).[13]

resources are to be used to deal with toxic residues. Marsh and Day[13] built a risk assessment process that divided risk assessment into four stages. They called their process model a checklist and it appears in Table 8.3.

Both the checklist and the process–model checklist rate each site by the same set of metrics. The difference between them is that the Marsh and Day checklist involves considerable research by experts. For example, the first item in the process–model checklist involves analyzing the toxicity of the five most hazardous substances on site. The following optional answers are provided:

- 0 = none
- 1 = low
- 2 = medium
- 3 = high
- 9 = no data/unknown

If formaldehyde is one of the substances, for example, Marsh and Day provide a table that rates formaldehyde as 3 in toxicity, 0 in persistence, 2 in ignitability, and 0 in reactivity. These numbers are summed to arrive at a toxicity rating of either "strong" or "weak." Similar assessments are made for exposure pathways, human exposures, and health outcomes. Each site will have a final score across all of these criteria. Then the Marsh and Day paper suggests alternative risk management strategies.

This process model requires investigators to obtain the data from the site before they can classify each into risk categories. It has several notable limitations. Break points between the risk categories are based on professional judgment; sites are placed into broad categories at each of the four steps; and some risk analysts are uncomfortable with semiquantitative groupings of risk and locations that depend upon professional judgment rather than being grounded in hard evidence. This means that judgmental errors, even by experts, can potentially place people at risk or unnecessarily worry them.

The U.S. Environmental Protection Agency (EPA) used a somewhat more complex semiquantitative model, the Hazard Ranking System prepared by the Mitre Corporation, to prioritize and then allocate billions of taxpayer dollars for the cleanup to thousands of eligible contaminated sites in the United States.[14] The logic of both the Marsh and Day and EPA approaches are transferable to brownfield and grayfield site cleanups when the threat to human health and safety is limited and there are many sites to rank. Therein, however, is the seed for concern. Even though these models can help decision-makers sort options across many locations into categories, can anything short of a site-specific analysis provide credible evidence of the degree of risk at a particular site?

When an individual site clearly has been identified as problematic by checklists and semiquantitative risk assessment tools, then a more focused site-specific approach is required. The U.S. Agency for Toxic Substances and Disease Registry (ATSDR) recently created a Web-based program to consider the impact of brownfield and land reuse on human health and safety.[15] The program is intended to allow health officials at the local and state levels, regulators, and developers to build a database that may be used to estimate human health effects of proposed development projects. The ATSDR tool requires the following:

- Historical, present, and possible future uses
- Community characteristics
- Selected land uses, facilities hosting seniors and children, and schools

The local user uses screens to input data, such as "Does the site attract children and pets?" and detailed information about the size of the site, its soil, and other structural information. It requests information about institutional controls (e.g., security, fencing, land use), a list of any violations, and land uses in the past, present, and possibly the future. Although the site is somewhat tedious to use, the data entry and checking tasks can be performed by a group of people.

The ATSDR tool requires users to think about likely exposure pathways (air, water, food, soil). It has internal estimates and multipliers and uses these to report ingestion and inhalation exposures, including 95 percent confidence limits, and reports on the quality of the input data. The tool requires Microsoft Access and local expertise for effective use. To minimize the frustration of false starts, we suggest inviting a speaker who has used the package to assess its suitability for a specific application.

Although this tool clearly has potential, we would like to see it applied in the field with realistic results rather than generic ones. By this we mean that when a redevelopment project is likely to costs tens of millions to more than a billion dollars to remediate, and when there are chances for major exposure scenarios, a more detailed risk assessment and management process should be considered beyond what might be available through this tool. We offer by way of further explanation the detailed risk assessment done in the Fernald case study.

Case Study: Reuse of the Fernald Nuclear Weapon Site

On July 16, 1945, the United States successfully tested the first nuclear weapon in New Mexico. In August 1945, it dropped nuclear weapons on two Japanese cities, Hiroshima and Nagasaki. The outcome was more than 100,000 killed, many injuries, and the destruction of tens of thousands of buildings. For the United States, the benefits arguably were a more rapid ending of the Pacific war without a need to invade Japan. The action may have saved well over a million people from being killed and injured. A massive amount has been written about the building, use, and consequences of using these weapons.[16–19]

What are often missed in public discussion are the human health, safety, and environmental legacies of the nuclear development effort in the United States after the war. To design, build, and test these weapons and the next generation of them, the United States created a nuclear factory with more than 100 sites. Sixteen sites are still being remediated. Former DOE Secretary Hazel O'Leary eloquently stated the moral commitment:

> The United States built the world's first atomic bomb to help win World War II and developed a nuclear arsenal to fight the Cold War. How we unleashed the fundamental power of the universe is one of the greatest stories of our era. It is a story of extraordinary challenges brilliantly met, a story of genius, teamwork industry, and courage.
>
> We are now embarked on another great challenge and a new national priority: refocusing the commitment to build the most powerful weapons on Earth toward the widespread environmental and safety problems at thousands of contaminated sites across the lands. We have a moral obligation to do no less, and we are committed to producing meaningful results. This is the honorable and challenging task of the Department's Environmental Management Program.[20]

Some of the legacy nuclear weapons sites are massive, well over 100 square miles. These will be in remediation for many decades to come: Hanford in eastern Washington State (about 590 square miles); Savannah River in Aiken, South Carolina, adjacent to the Savannah River (about 300 square miles); and the Idaho National Laboratory site

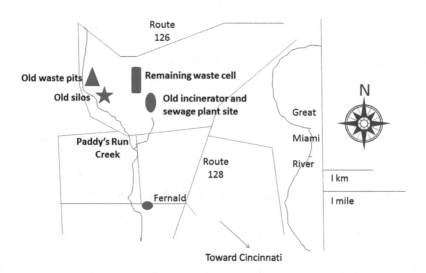

Note: Locations are not to scale in order to emphasize key sites, and selected routes are shown. Site is about 18 miles from Cincinnati.

Figure 8.2. Fernald Site Elements

(about 890 square miles), west of Idaho Falls.[10,21] During the period 1989 to 2013, the DOE spent more than $150 billion to remediate more than 100 sites, about $6 billion a year. Sixteen sites remain in their portfolio, and the estimated cost of cleanup of these is $200 billion to $300 billion. More than 70 percent of the cost, more than $200 billion, is estimated to be spent at the three locations in Washington State, South Carolina, and Idaho. These are unprecedented cleanup and risk management expenditures, the most costly environmental management cleanup costs in the world.[22–24]

Compared with several of those sites, the Fernald site has been a modest project (Figure 8.2). Located about 18 miles northwest of Cincinnati in Crosby, Ohio, the 1,050-acre site was called the Fernald Feed Materials Production Center and was part of the nationwide nuclear weapons production factory from 1951 through 1988.[21]

The Fernald site was originally designed as a large factory complex, with tall stacks and waste ponds. The site took uranium ore that was already concentrated and produced target elements for nuclear reactors and other elements needed to produce nuclear weapons. Paddy's Run, a very small stream, flows southward along the western boundary of the site. The Great Miami River lies about a mile away and flows south, meandering several times near the eastern border of the site. The entire site overlies the Great Miami aquifer.

The federal government chose the Fernald site because it had military nuclear reactors relatively nearby in Oak Ridge (Tennessee) and Savannah River (South Carolina). Fernald could also receive uranium imports through major ports in New York, New York, and New Orleans, Louisiana. The site itself was relatively easy to build on. There was a large labor force about 20 miles away in Cincinnati, and a large aquifer under the site could be tapped for water. Chemical and metallurgical processes were used at multiple facilities on the site. The Sampling Plant took samples of the incoming ore. The Refinery and Denitrification Plant concentrated the ore and transformed it into more refined products. In the process, liquid nitrogen dioxide fumes and nitric acid were emitted into the air. The refined material was pumped, reacted, and moved again for additional processing, which led to periodic spills and boil overs.

From an engineering perspective, the plant produced materials that the federal government needed to produce the tens of thousands of nuclear weapons used to pursue the Cold War.[20,21,25-27] During Fernald's production years, radioactive material was released from three main sources. One was from material stored in two large silos (K-65 silos), which held waste contaminated with radium. The second source was waste burned in incinerators. Waste buried in storage pits was a third, and liquid radioactive waste ran off and formed a groundwater plume that moved in- and off-site into the Great Miami aquifer.[28,29] Typical of a factory complex, as processes were improved, old facilities were mothballed, and new ones were created. When operations are focused around enriched uranium, it is more than reasonable for the local population to be concerned about how facilities age and transition their processes.

After three decades of operations, Fernald received a great deal of negative attention in 1984, when the public learned that the facility had been releasing uranium dust into the air and that leaks into the ground were common. This caused concern about the Great Miami aquifer, which also happens to be a sole source of water for many people in the larger region. Furthermore, concern was raised when an employee was found dead on the site, and a conspiracy theory quickly developed that he was murdered to cover up exposures. The death of Dave Bocks was covered on the show *Unsolved Mysteries* on June 19, 1984.[30] By watching that show, surely many became concerned about what was going on at the Fernald site.

Shortly afterward, 14,000 Ohio residents filed a class action suit against the site. Writing for the *New York Times*, Noble summarized the litany of issues.[31] The DOE was accused of allowing uranium and waste to leak from the site. The reporter emphasized that government officials publicly acknowledged for the first time in court that they "knew full well" that the plant would emit uranium and other substances into water supplies and the air. Former site managers acknowledged that they had insufficient resources to manage health and safety issues. An elected official asserted that the DOE was in effect waging chemical warfare against local residents.

Fernald became even more infamous when Ohio sued the federal government. Reporting on the case in the *Villanova Environmental Law Journal*, May includes the following statement in the first sentence: "the federal government itself has earned the reputation as one of the nation's worst polluters."[32] May then proceeded to explain that the Fernald case shows that the federal government claims sovereign immunity as a reason for not responding to suits from other government branches. Fernald was a sufficiently distressing case that merited interest by investigative reporters from *60 Minutes* and *20/20*.[33]

Risk Assessment

Given the human health and safety risks and the existence of federal legislation that mandated more formal risk studies, there was little to no chance that the public was going to settle for a checklist, or even a semiquantitative risk assessment of Fernald. In 1988, Congress called for the Centers for Disease Control and Prevention (CDC) to conduct an epidemiologic study of human health outcomes in the Fernald area. The CDC recognized that such a study would produce meaningless results unless an exposure assessment was completed as part of a larger risk assessment.

Using mathematical air and water models, the CDC completed a risk assessment in two phases. The first focused on lung cancer[28] and the second on kidney, female breast, and bone cancer, and leukemia.[29] The study area was a circular area with a radius of 10 kilometers (6.2 miles) around the center of the site. Analysts estimated that 43,000 to 53,000 people lived in that circular area during the operating years between 1951 and 1988. Given that prevailing winds are to the northeast, the area was further subdivided into 12 cardinal compass areas. In the case of lung cancer deaths, the risk assessors estimated the population dose, the risk of dying from estimated doses, and the number of residents who received selected doses during the study period.

As the semiquantitative approaches described earlier were not applicable to the Fernald case, the analysts from the CDC used available data to estimate the median number of additional cancers within a 90 percent acceptable range. Lung cancer was the most important health risk because of airborne emissions of uranium. Secondarily, analysts estimated bone, kidney, leukemia, and female breast cancers associated with contaminated drinking water and air emissions.

Table 8.4 shows the expected number of deaths from the CDC's risk assessment. The results estimated that Fernald would add 1 to 12 percent more cancer deaths to the area, the vast majority of which would be lung cancer among males who also were smokers. The additional deaths were calculated based on an additional dose of 0.45 sieverts with a range of 0.12 to 1.74 sieverts. A sievert is a unit of ionizing radiation dose where 1 sievert = 100 rem of gamma radiation. Most of this exposure would be from breathing radon decay products, especially to the east of site, which is where the prevailing winds would take the emissions. Most of the fatal cases were allotted to the period before the year 2000 because of the aging of the population and because emissions controls were placed on two silos in 1979. In other words, risk assessors were estimating that there would be much less airborne risk in the future.

Table 8.4. Cancer Deaths Estimated for Fernald Studies

Population	Background Median (90% credibility interval)	Fernald-Related Median (90% credibility interval)
Lung cancer, entire population	2601 (2257-3014)	85 (25-309)
Lung cancer, ever smokers	2302 (1997-2666)	65 (19-238)
Lung cancer, males	1692 (1496-1978)	49 (14-187)
Breast cancer, females	2296 (1945-2717)	1 (0-3)
Bone cancer	32 (27-38)	1 (0-4)
Kidney cancer	367 (311-435)	1 (0-4)
Leukemia	367 (311-435)	5 (3-23)

Source: Based on Centers for Disease Control and Prevention.[28,29]
Note: Background includes the estimated number of deaths without the effect of Fernald exposures.

The risk models used in the CDC's analyses were based on exposures of uranium mineworkers and of survivors from the two atom bombs dropped on Japan. These were the best data available, but conditions at Fernald and other nuclear facilities were not the same. For non-lung cancers, it was assumed that all vegetables eaten by those with the most exposures were contaminated, as was all the milk, beef, chicken, egg, and fish that the victims ate. This assumption demonstrates how risk assessors sometimes tend to be unrealistically conservative when estimating risks. The CDC estimated the expected number of deaths from cancers (background level data) from cancer registry records and followed the normal practice of assuming that lung cancer is much more likely among smokers. The assessors found the vast majority of cancers were lung cancers occurring among current and former smokers. Did an increase of 1 to 12 percent in cancers justify the expenditures of billions of dollars on risk management? Clearly, the federal government decided that it was.

Risk Management

As the DOE was severely criticized and sued by the local population surrounding Fernald, it became obvious that a minimum risk management effort was not going to be tolerated. The site was a Superfund site, which meant that the DOE was subject to multiple federal legal requirements, including community participation. A major issue for the DOE was that it had little credibility and the chances were high that not only the public but also senior elected officials would challenge whatever decision it made. A constructive way of approaching a mutually agreeable resolution was to commit to trying to return the site to pre-DOE status at an estimated cost of $7 billion to $10 billion. However, even these expensive options would have been opposed because of some of the environmental implications.

Because of the complexity of the situation at Fernald, the DOE and its partners turned to a collaborative process aided by the work of a national-level committee. The Federal Facilities Environmental Restoration Dialogue Committee (FFERDC) was organized by the EPA to discuss how federal agencies (primarily DOE, Department of Defense, EPA, and other agencies with expensive challenges) should allocate limited cleanup funds.[21] The FFERDC issued a set of recommendations that were adopted as a guide by federal agencies. More than a decade later, at a meeting chaired by the first author to discuss allocation of the DOE's environmental management resources, DOE officials prominently displayed a copy of the FFERDC report.[21,22] A key message from the report is that human health and safety risk was the primary factor driving funding allocation but that other factors had to be considered. The addition of these factors has since become known as the "risk plus other factors" approach. These other factors include the following:

- Cultural, social, and economic factors, notably environmental justice
- Long- and short-term ecological impacts, especially degradation of resource value and, hence, use
- Land use decisions, especially as these impact the economic health of the area
- Acceptability of the proposed action to regulators, and the public
- Incorporation of the views of Tribal Nations into project designs
- Life cycle costs
- Importance of reducing infrastructure and operation–maintenance costs
- Availability of new technologies
- Legal and statutory requirements
- Cost and effectiveness of proposed actions
- Availability of funding
- Practical considerations, such as accomplishing projects and working on remediation projects without hindering others' activities

The lawsuit brought by Fernald citizens against the DOE was settled in 1989, and the immediate concerns of the local public were addressed by offering biannual health monitoring and financial compensation. However, the DOE's credibility was shaky, and the DOE and State of Ohio agreed that a citizens' advisory board would be a good choice for gaining input on priorities and rebuilding trust. The FFERDC suggested establishing advisory boards, and the Fernald Board became a model that the DOE adopted not only for the site but also for other DOE sites that have since been closed (e.g., Mound and Rocky Flats).

A key part of the success enjoyed by the Fernald collaboration was that Dr. Eula Bingham, a professor at the University of Cincinnati, was hired to find and then interview candidates to serve on the advisory board. Bingham, with degrees in chemistry, biology, and zoology, served as director of the U.S. Occupational Safety and Health

Administration from 1972 through 1976 under President Carter. Her strong academic record as a scientist combined with her administrative experience made her a highly credible leader. This allowed her to identify and consider who should be part of the advisory board and then persuade strong individuals to serve. Her recommendations were accepted, and the Fernald Citizens Task Force (hereafter called Task Force) was established in 1993. John Applegate, a law professor at the University of Cincinnati, was the Task Force's first chair. Applegate added additional prestige because of his scholarly and legal experiences.[3]

As per the suggestions of the FFERDC report, a diverse committee of up to 14 and alternates was appointed. The majority of Task Force members worked at the site or lived near it. The rest represented specific interests and skill sets. In addition, four members were appointed ex-officio representing the DOE, the federal EPA, the Ohio EPA, and the ATSDR. The responsible parties (as defined under the Comprehensive Environmental Response, Compensation, and Liability Act [CERCLA] or Superfund), the DOE, and regulators asked the Task Force to address four issues:

- Preferred future use for the site
- Allowable residual risk and appropriate remediation levels
- Disposal options for onsite wastes
- Remediation priorities

With regard to the first committee charge, the Task Force recognized that they needed a professional facilitator with technical expertise. Douglas Sarno of Phoenix Environmental served in this role for almost 13 years. The key focus of the group was to determine the preferred future use and employ that idea as the basis for remediation. They also created explicit goals, rules, and procedures, and specifics such as length of term, chair, and vice-chair positions. The Task Force adopted the principle that meetings were to be open to the public (>100 attended some meetings), and the public would have a comment period.[25] A great deal of Task Force work was focused around understanding the attributes of the site, the waste, and community information such as preferences and values. DOE staff, site contractors, regulators, and others provided briefings and data. From a strategic perspective, not only did these sessions help Task Force members understand the site and the community but the process also built trust among the members, as well as with those providing information to the Task Force.

The Task Force incorporated *FutureSite* into some of their meetings, a game that allowed the group to more deeply explore the relationships between future land use and remediation. The game had chips, cards, and other elements of a board game and was intended to help Task Force members understand human health and safety risks, costs, and other risk management decisions that needed to be made. Applegate and Sarno described the details of the game[34] and there are other more detailed descriptions and illustrations embedded in the Fernald Citizens Advisory Board records.[25]

After considerable discussion and debate, the Task Force made decisions that surprised many. They realized that to completely remove all the waste would require a massive amount of soil removal from the area and the shipment of a large amount of waste from Ohio to Nevada (the only location that could accept it). The decision was to remove the most dangerous material (about 20 percent) that threatened the aquifer and leave a great deal of the less hazardous wastes (about 80 percent) that could be managed on site in a large hill surrounded by a buffer zone to protect the structure (see Figure 8.2, the area marked "remaining waste cell"), especially the cap, against intruders. Removal of uranium from the aquifer was a high priority and is ongoing.

Before the cleanup, the operating site looked like a typical chemical and oil industrial facility with towers, pits, pipes, and the tops of tanks, open lagoons, and intersecting roads. After closure and remediation, it is open space, with prairies and upland forest. There are visible walking paths and an educational center, along with a hill along the east side of the site. That hill is not accessible to visitors as it contains about 80 percent of the remaining waste. If you did not know what the site had been used for, it blends in with the surrounding farmscape, except the surrounding area is primarily square farm plots without a hill that does not seem to belong there.

The DOE and the regulators accepted the Task Force recommendations, albeit the process had some bumps. After some members of the Task Force left, the group was reconstituted as the Fernald Citizens Advisory Board (CAB). It took on additional challenging risk management decisions. For example, how was the most hazardous material shipped off site? Risk assessments and management analyses were done, and the CAB took the position that rail should be used as much as possible to reduce risk and be more cost-effective. Initially the DOE's contractors and the DOE itself was skeptical, but they changed their views as the analyses were done, presented, and discussed.

The CAB examined the cleanup of the two contaminated silos. After much debate, the idea that the nuclear waste was to be vitrified (mixed with molten glass in a large stainless steel cylinder) for long-term storage was abandoned because of the composition of the waste. Although the CAB did not achieve unanimous support for the decision, it approved placing the material in cement. The CAB persuaded the DOE to add a fixing agent to the waste to prevent it from becoming airborne and worked with the DOE to transfer waste off the site to locations that originally were not considered acceptable.

When the remediation process started, the initial estimate was that it would take 25 years to complete. With strong advocacy by the CAB, the schedule was reduced to 10 years. These two decisions and several others required the CAB to take strong positions and persuade the DOE and the regulators that these were the most effective decisions. Part of the effort was focused on creating an image of the site as an asset rather than a local liability. The site was given a new image as an education center, with a nature preserve and public walking trails. The education center hosts an exhibit on the history of the site, with testimony by former site workers, officials, and residents. It is intended to make sure that the local community is vigilant about the site.[25,27]

When the first author visited the site, it reminded him of trips to an old U.S. Civil War battlefield or similar sites in Europe and China.

Uranium in the aquifer has been removed by pump and treat, and thousands of tons of low-level waste will be stored on site for thousands of years. Yet, while accepting that reality, the focus of the CAB was on the site becoming a recreation facility. Design charrettes were quite important to guide the group. Part of the plan required the DOE and the regulators to agree to implement legally binding institutional controls, including that the DOE would manage the remaining waste cell (see Figure 8.2) and the surrounding green space into perpetuity.

Arguably, without the Task Force and the CAB, the DOE would have taken a quarter of a century and spent more than $10 billion to manage this site. Instead, about $4.4 billion was spent over a decade to create a sustainably protective engineered system supported by legal agreements, institutional controls, and a public education and recreation center. The three tools described in this chapter were pivotal in the process.

Final Thoughts

Had this not been a DOE site, or another organization with deep financial pockets and with a moral and legal commitment to clean up, the application of these expensive tools might not have been possible. Laws and regulations required some of the tools. The cleanup was managed under a variety of statutes, but CERCLA was the most important. Accordingly, Fernald was going to involve risk assessment, some form of cost–benefit and/or effectiveness analyses, exposure assessment, epidemiology, and some form of public process, although not necessarily as much collaborative problem solving as happened. Fernald is a case in which federal, state, and local decision-makers realized that an acceptable engineered solution was not going to suffice. While many tools were part of the process (e.g., environmental impact statements, social network analysis, benefit–cost analysis, and regional economic impacts), Fernald required active citizen participation. The Fernald case utilized a classical collaborative process model that was grounded in good science and planning, as have been other cases reported in the literature.[35,36]

References

1. Gray B. *Collaborating: Finding Common Ground for Multiparty Problems.* San Francisco, CA: Jossey-Bass Publishers; 1989.

2. Hartnett T. *Consensus-Oriented Decision-Making: The CODM Model for Facilitating Groups to Widespread Agreement*. Gabriola Island, BC: New Society Publishers; 2011.

3. Applegate JS. Beyond the usual suspects: The use of citizens advisory boards in environmental decisionmaking. *Indiana Law J*. 1998;73(3):903–957.

4. Saint S, Lawson J. *Rules for Reaching Consensus: A Modern Approach to Decision Making*. Amsterdam, The Netherlands; San Diego, CA: Pfeiffer & Co; 1994.

5. Sarkissian W, Perlgut D, eds. *The Community Participation Handbook: Resources for Public Involvement in the Planning Process*. 2nd ed. Murdoch, WA: Murdoch University, Institute for Sustainability and Technology Policy; 2005.

6. Susskind LE, McKearnen S, Thomas-Lamar J. *The Consensus Building Handbook: A Comprehensive Guide to Reaching Agreement*. Thousand Oaks, CA: SAGE Publications; 1999.

7. Linstone H, Turoff M. The Delphi Method techniques and applications. 2002. Available at: https://pdfs.semanticscholar.org/8634/72a67f5bdc67e4782306efd883fca23e3a3d.pdf. Accessed February 26, 2016.

8. Idea Rating Sheets: a simple tool to help large groups find agreement. Available at: http://www.idearatingsheets.org. Accessed February 29, 2016.

9. Lindsey G, Todd J, Hayter S, Ellis P. *A Handbook for Planning and Conducting Charrettes for High Performance Projects*. 2009. Available at: http://www.nrel.gov/docs/fy03osti/33425.pdf. Accessed February 26, 2016.

10. Greenberg M. *Nuclear Waste Management, Nuclear Power, and Energy Choices: Public Preferences, Perceptions, and Trust*. New York, NY: Springer Publishers; 2012.

11. Greenberg M, Belnay G, Cesanek W, Neuman N, Shepherd G. *A Primer on Industrial Environmental Impact*. New Brunswick, NJ: Center for Urban Policy Research, Rutgers University; 1979.

12. Greenberg G, Burger J, Gochfeld M, et al. End-state land uses, sustainably protective systems, and risk management: a challenge for remediation and multigenerational stewardship. *Remediation*. 2005;16(1):91–105.

13. Marsh G, Day R. A model standardized risk assessment protocol for use with hazardous waste sites. *Environ Health Perspect*. 1991;90:199–208.

14. National Research Council. *Ranking Hazardous-Waste Sites for Remedial Action*. Washington, DC: National Academies Press; 1994.

15. Agency for Toxic Substances and Disease Registry. ATSDR brownfield and land reuse health initiative—ATSDR site tool. Available at: http://www.atsdr.cdc.gov/sites/brownfields/site_inventory.html. Accessed February 26, 2016.

16. Cooke S. *In Mortal Hands: A Cautionary History of the Nuclear Age*. Collingswood, Australia: Black Inc; 2009.

17. Groves L. *Now It Can Be Told: The Story of the Manhattan Project*. New York, NY: Da Capo Press; 1983.

18. Schwartz S, ed. *Atomic Audit: The Costs and Consequences of US Nuclear Weapons Since 1940*. Washington, DC: Brookings; 2011.

19. Teller E, Brown A. *The Legacy of Hiroshima*. Garden City, NY: Doubleday; 1962.

20. *Closing the Circle on the Splitting of the Atom*. Washington, DC: US Department of Energy; 1995.

21. *Charting a Course for the Future: A Report on Firm Preparedness*. Washington, DC: US Department of Energy; 1996.

22. A review of the use of risk-informed management in the cleanup program for former defense nuclear sites, report prepared from U.S. Senate and House of Representatives Committees on Appropriations (August 2015). Washington, DC: Omnibus Risk Review Committee; 2015.

23. US Department of Energy Office of the Chief Financial Officer. FY 2014 Budget Justification. Available at: http://energy.gov/cfo/downloads/fy-2014-budget-justification. Accessed February 29, 2016.

24. US Department of Energy Office of the Chief Financial Officer. Department of Energy FY 2015 Congressional Budget Request: environmental management, DOE/CF-0100 Volume 5. 2014. Available at: http://energy.gov/sites/prod/files/2014/12/f19/EM_FY2015_Congressional_Budget_Request.pdf. Accessed February 26, 2016.

25. Fernald Citizens Advisory Board. History and accomplishments of the Fernald Citizens Advisory Board, 1993–2006. Participedia. 2013. Available at: http://www.lm.doe.gov/land/sites/oh/FernaldCAB/FCABHistory/index.html. Accessed February 26, 2016.

26. US Department of Energy Office of Legacy Management. Fernald community archive. Available at: http://www.lm.doe.gov/Fernald/Meetings.aspx. Accessed February 26, 2016.

27. US Department of Energy Office of Legacy Management. Fernald Preserve, Ohio. 2016. Available at: http://www.lm.doe.gov/fernald/Sites.aspx. Accessed February 26, 2016.

28. Fernald risk assessment project, estimation of the impact of the former Feed Material Production Center (FMPC) on lung cancer mortality in the surrounding community. Washington, DC: Centers for Disease Control and Prevention; 1998.

29. Fernald risk assessment project, phase II. Screening level estimates of the lifetime risk of developing kidney cancer, female breast cancer, bone cancer, leukemia. Washington, DC: Centers for Disease Control and Prevention; 2000.

30. Dave Bocks. Unsolved Mysteries. 1994. Available at: http://unsolvedmysteries.wikia.com/wiki/Dave_Bocks. Accessed February 26, 2016.

31. Noble K. U.S., for decades, let uranium leak at weapon plant. *New York Times*. October 15, 1988. Available at: http://www.nytimes.com/1988/10/15/us/us-for-decades-let-uranium-leak-at-weapon-plant.html. Accessed February 26, 2016.

32. May G. *United States Department of Energy v. Ohio* and the Federal Facility Compliance Act of 1992: the Supreme Court forces a hazardous compromise in CWA and RCRA enforcement against federal agencies. *Villanova Environ Law J.* 1993;4(2):363–393.

33. US Department of Energy Fernald closure project. The end of secrecy. Available at: http://www.lm.doe.gov/land/sites/oh/fernald_orig/50th/secr.htm. Accessed September 16, 2016.

34. Applegate J, Sarno D. Futuresite: an environmental remediation game-simulation. *Simul Gaming.* 1997;28(1):13–27.

35. Beierle TC. Using social goals to evaluate public participation in environmental decisions. *Rev Policy Res.* 2005;16(3–4):75–103.

36. Branch KM, Bradbury JA. Comparison of DOE and army advisory boards: application of a conceptual framework for evaluating public participation in environmental risk decision making. *Policy Stud J.* 2006;34(4):723–754.

9

EVALUATING A PROPOSED MAJOR REGIONAL ASSET

The context for this chapter is that influential actors want to build facilities or add programs that they believe to be important and consistent with both their organizations' goals and a strong regional economy. They are boosters who have a tendency to overstate the benefits of what they want to achieve and deemphasize any problems that might occur. Other community members oppose the project, and they will voice objections and take a not-in-my-backyard (NIMBY) stance. This scenario has played out in hundreds of places in reaction to proposals for new or expanded airports, roads, rail lines, bridges and tunnels, factories, electric power generation facilities, waste management sites, large building complexes, cell towers, prisons, and many others.[1-6]

As pressure from proponents and opponents builds, public health practitioners and planners are required to express their views, typically about how to mitigate impacts or how to craft a case for or against the project. Every one of the tools reviewed in Chapters 5 through 8 can be part of their toolkit. Based on our experience, the following would be most likely: checklists, collaborative problem solving, environmental justice analysis, focus groups and surveys, risk assessment and risk management, social network analysis, and spatial environmental data analysis.

This chapter introduces, highlights, and illustrates three tools that will be or should be part of the effort involved to understand these projects:

- Environmental impact statements
- Regional economic impact analysis
- Benefit and cost analysis

We demonstrate the usefulness of these tools in two case studies: the building of the Denver International Airport (DIA) and a proposed but not constructed liquefied natural gas (LNG) plant at Sparrows Point, Maryland.

Environmental Impact Statements

The National Environmental Policy Act (NEPA), signed into law by President Richard Nixon on January 1, 1970, is the most emulated U.S. law, with more than 100 countries having a adopted a version of it. Public Law 91-190 was intended to "create and maintain conditions under which man and nature can exist in productive harmony and fulfill the social, economic and other requirements of present and future generations."[7]

Preparation of an environmental impact statement (EIS) is part of NEPA legal requirements. Before reviewing the details involved in preparing an EIS, we begin by underscoring two common misunderstandings about the EIS process that will become apparent as you read this chapter:

Misunderstanding #1: The EIS is a decision-making document.

It is not. Rather, the EIS is a decision-informing tool. Decisions are made by the secretary of the federal department overseeing the permitting process for the project. Their decision may or may not be consistent with EIS findings.

Misunderstanding #2: The EIS focuses on a selected set of key environmental outcomes.

In reality, an EIS tends to be encyclopedic. This is because analysts do not want their proposals rejected because they forgot to include an issue that may later be challenged in U.S. courts. Thus, an EIS document may include several volumes and thousands of pages.

These two misunderstandings show how NEPA has fallen short of becoming the Magna Carta for the environment that many hoped it would be. Despite the legislation's shortcomings, Section 102c of NEPA requires all federal agencies to prepare an EIS on proposed legislation and other major federal actions that could significantly affect the quality of the human environment. This requires substantial analysis, outreach, and documentation.[8-10]

Federal agencies prepare EISs because they are required to do so by federal law for the following kinds of projects: those supported by federal money or federal legislative proposals. They may also prepare an EIS when significant changes to federal government policies and operations are anticipated, and they require an EIS for projects for which they must issue federal permits, licenses, and other approvals.

Paraphrasing the legislation, regulations, and court interpretations of NEPA, federal agencies involved in any of the types of projects listed in the previous paragraph are required to

- Assess their environmental impact.
- Indicate any adverse environmental impacts that cannot be avoided if the proposal is implemented.
- Provide alternative actions (a preferred alternative, alternatives to it, and no-action).
- Explain the relationship between local short-term uses of the environment and long-term productivity.
- Indicate irreversible and resource commitments if the project is implemented.

Not every action requires a full EIS. Agencies may request a waiver of the EIS requirement on the basis of analyses that show little chance of environmental impact. This
would allow them to prepare a shorter environmental assessment that follows the EIS
format but is likely to be only 5 to 10 percent of the length of a full EIS.[10]

Requests for exemptions with shorter EISs have been challenged, leading to good case
law on what constitutes "major" and "significant" actions or proposals and what constitutes an "adequate" EIS.

EISs almost always include a multidisciplinary team that seeks to accomplish the
following[10]:

- Describe the existing environment.
- Describe a preferred alternative, one or more other alternatives, and a no-action
  alternative.
- Describe the impact of each alternative on the environment.
- Explain why one alternative is preferred.
- Describe steps to mitigate any more environmental impacts.

To complete these tasks the multidisciplinary team will likely take the following organizational actions[10,11]:

1. Hold internal and open public meetings to understand concerns, including
   receiving letters and other communications from the public.
2. Review, collect, and assess available data to address impacts.
3. Identify data gaps and collect information to fill them.
4. Prepare plan for the EIS and format for the final EIS.
5. Prepare a preliminary EIS document and circulate it to partners.
6. Get feedback and prepare a draft EIS (DEIS).
7. Get feedback and prepare a final EIS (FEIS) for external review.
8. If needed, prepare supplemental EISs to address new issues.

Federal agencies are responsible for EISs, but the work is delegated to proponents of the
project or to private companies that specialize in preparing EISs. Some states have their
own EIS process, as do some local governments. We recommend California's EIS process
as a state model[12] and San Francisco's as a local one.[13] The state and local versions are
shorter and tend to place greater emphasis on human health and issues such as housing.
You can determine if your state or local government has an EIS requirement by checking
their Web sites.

Earlier we noted that some people expect decision-makers to follow the conclusions
of the EIS and expect an EIS will focus on only a few possible key impacts, neither of
which is true. There are also other criticisms of the EIS process. One is that the federal
legislation does not require an EIS process of private organizations unless they receive
government funds or require federal government approvals. Most large infrastructure

projects are required to complete EISs because they do need federal support. Among the most often heard criticisms is that the EIS process takes too long to complete and costs too much. This has led to efforts to change the process, limit its use, and allow for shorter environmental assessments. There is also political pressure on agencies to issue declarations that an EIS is not needed because there will be no major environmental impacts.

On the other hand, the EIS provides a great deal of information that can be used to inform decisions, sometimes leading to cancellation or alterations in plans for major projects. We have seen some proposals stopped because they could not make it through the EIS process and others scaled down to a more acceptable size.[10,11] EISs are public documents and the basic data they develop can be used in studies that may be unrelated to the specific project for which they were designed. As such, EISs have become de facto land use planning for U.S. national and regional-scale projects.

A U.S. Government Accountability Office (GAO) study in 2014[14] reported difficulty in determining how many EISs have been done. For the period 2001 to 2008, the GAO estimated that about 129 were done annually. In 2011, the agency estimated only 94. In contrast to the GAO findings, we searched for draft or final EIS documents that were submitted for the period January 1970 through November 1977 and found 8,500 of them, or more than 1,000 per year. In fact, almost 2,000 were submitted in 1971 alone, and submissions have steadily fallen off since then as the GAO report indicates. Full EIS reports are characterized by the GAO as high-profile, complex, and expensive (costing $250,000 to $2 million). About 95 percent of proposals that might require an EIS are excused from preparing one or they are required only to prepare a shorter version. In the early 1970s, the first author proclaimed that NEPA's EIS requirement was a "full employment act" for his students. Today, he tells them they might be lucky if they get to work on one. They are far more likely to have to consult one or to evaluate several.

Regional Economic Impact Analysis

When a new airport is built, we know that architects, engineers, and construction workers are all involved in building the facilities. Once built, pilots, aircraft maintenance staff, on-flight assistants, guards, building and maintenance workers, and many others will be employed providing services to passengers. People located off-site will be employed to provide supplies and services to the airport. Some of the money and benefits that airport and off-site workers earn will be used to create jobs for local retailers, wholesalers, and many others. The expenditures will be taxed and the taxes used to hire police, firefighters, school teachers, and many others. In other words, the money moves through the economy, creating new income, jobs, and tax revenues.

Regional economic impact tools estimate how many dollars and jobs are created when something new is added or rebuilt. The tools take into account how many tax

Table 9.1. Desirable Attributes of Regional Economic Models

Attribute
• Estimate direct, indirect, and induced impacts of a project measured as gross regional product, income, jobs, unemployment, migration, and taxes.
• Estimate local-, regional- (multicounty), state-, national-, and international-level impacts.
• Estimate short-term (monthly, then quarterly), intermediate (annually for two to five years), and long-term (annually for five years or more).
• Estimate the impact of strategic investments in expanding infrastructure, resilience, and sustainability.
• Isolate economic impacts on already disadvantaged populations (poor, isolated, and impaired).

Source: Based on Greenberg et al. (2007).[15]

dollars are generated, and some have the capacity to estimate migration into and out of the area. Regional economic impact models are also used to determine the impacts of storms, earthquakes, wars, and other hazard events on regional economies. They can also be used to estimate the impacts of investing to rebuild in devastated areas. A good regional economic impact model should have all or at least some of the attributes found in Table 9.1.

Econometric Models

Econometric models are a set of equations that connect national, state, and local capital, labor, income, taxes, spending, and other elements of the economy. For example, if we know that about 10 percent of salary increases are spent on durable good purchases, then we can estimate how much the population will spend on new cars, televisions, and refrigerators.[15-17]

The equations are typically based on 25 to 30 years of historical records. In other words, econometric models are grounded in recent history. If the recent past is a good representation of the near-term future, then an econometric model will produce good economic impact estimates. However, if there is a sudden change in the economy, then econometric-based estimates will produce misleading results.

The complexity of econometric models can vary. The first author, for example, has used an econometric model for the State of New Jersey that includes 300 equations. This model was used along with one of about half that size for a portion of New York State to evaluate the greater metropolitan area. Larger models are more desirable than smaller ones because they pinpoint potentially important portions of the regional economy that might be otherwise overlooked.

A big advantage of econometric models is that they produce annual, semiannual, and even monthly economic estimates. Accordingly, the impact of a new facility can be measured as the difference between the forecasted economic growth with and without the new facility. The major weakness of econometric models is reliance on relationships observed in the recent past.

Input–Output Models

Input–output (I–O) models are the second major classical economic modeling alternative.[15,18] I–O models are massive spreadsheets of transactions within an economy. Suppose my town is going to build a new school. It will need land, architects, engineering, and environmental services, as well as concrete, steel, desks, boards, computers, teachers, and many other products and services. Analysis with an I–O model starts with the proposed design and uses the I–O spreadsheet to estimate the direct product and service purchases required to build and operate the facility. In turn, these transactions lead to additional purchases of goods and services throughout the economy (multiplier effects).

A major advantage of an I–O model is the ability to identify the flow of goods and services not only on site but also in the surrounding areas. A typical I–O analysis provides an estimate of the economic impacts, but it does not provide an estimate of the impacts for a specific period of time. Hence, it is not unusual for econometric models, which are times series tools, to be used together with I–O analysis models.

Both I–O and econometric models have the same limitations. That is, if the economy changes during the period of interest, the models can produce misleading results. Furthermore, because I–O data matrices have massive data requirements, they are not refreshed as often as econometric ones. This means the transaction matrices of an I–O model can become stale and produce inaccurate results in a dynamic economy. Consider the new school example. Now suppose a new type of classroom furniture becomes available and is preferred by the school board. The original estimates of impacts produced by the I–O model will differ from what actually happens when the school opens.

Overall, econometric and I–O models have the distinct advantage of being known to many who have studied in economics departments, business schools, or in economic geography or regional science programs. Each model produces valuable insights when the economy is not substantially in flux. The results are estimates of income, production, jobs, taxes, and migration.

Computable General Equilibrium and Regional Economic Models

Analysts have developed several approaches to adjust for the limitations of econometric and I–O models. One of these is a computable general equilibrium model

(CGE).[19,20] At the heart of the CGE model is an I–O model. When the economy is changing, analysts add modeling elements that assume the economy will shift to more efficient production processes. For example, less-water-demanding processes will be assumed during a drought. These changes are reflected in labor, capital, and other transactions in the economy. Of course, there is no guarantee that the CGE model will capture the changes. However, logically, it will capture some and hopefully the most important ones.

Regional Economic Models (REMI) offers an approach to overcome some of the limitations of the classical modeling approaches.[21,22] REMI includes interrelationships among income, wages, employment, prices, and other elements similar to those in econometric models. It also includes relationships among states and/or groups of regions with regard to interregional trade and migration among places in response to economic change. For example, if we build a new airport in one state, REMI can assess the potential economic impact on airports in adjacent areas.

The major limitations of CGE and REMI are their lack of familiarity to analysts and users. There are also the issues of significant added complexity and the additional time and cost involved in using these models. While a group of experts has begun to use CGE and REMI to estimate regional economic impacts, the models add an additional element of complexity in application, and interpretation of the results is difficult. Some of the new economic models, in fact, have been criticized as being black boxes that do not produce understandable results for decision-makers.

Regional economic modeling is not for the faint of heart. As an example, the second case study in this chapter, LNG exports, uses elements of all four of the models discussed in this chapter. The reader will see how the models provide estimates that depend upon a set of assumptions that may or may not be true. As a result, the models will provide results that are different enough to lead to different policy choices.

Benefit and Cost Analysis

Benefit and cost analysis (BCA), or cost and benefit analysis, is a process for estimating and comparing the economic benefits and costs of a proposed project or program.[23-27] A thorough BCA will include economic, social, health, environmental, and other elements of a proposed action measured in dollars or another currency. In addition, these costs will be estimated for the expected life of the project. For example, if a new dam is proposed, we want to know what value is associated with the amount of electricity that would be generated, recreational opportunities that would be created, and flood control benefits, among others. The costs of building the dam include concrete, steel, and labor, which are obvious ones, but also less obvious ones such as loss of land that is now beneath the dam and injuries to workers who construct the dam.

Like the EIS process, BCA has a standard set of analytical steps, which include the following:

- List alternative projects.
- Compile a list of interested parties, including those who will use the project, those who will build and operate the facilities, and others who will be indirectly impacted (e.g., lose their land or access to their land).
- Identify a set of metrics to use, including metrics for benefits and costs that are able to value subjective attributes, such as of the value that some people attach to the view of area without the dam.
- Estimate benefits and costs over the life cycle of the project.
- Convert all benefits and costs into a single currency.
- Apply a discount rate to account for the changing value of the project over time (the discount rate is the interest rate that the federal government charges banks to borrow capital).
- Calculate the net present value of the proposed project and other options.
- Conduct sensitivity analysis around the estimated values to account for uncertainty.

Assuming the estimates are deemed credible and politically acceptable, the project with the highest ratio of benefits to costs would be approved. In essence, a sound BCA expresses the utilitarian economic value of the policy for society as a whole.

The BCA process is criticized for many of the same reasons as the EIS one. Detractors argue that analysts rely too heavily on selected previous projects that are not relevant to the one being proposed. Despite the quantitative expression of the results (benefit-to-cost ratio), opponents charge that proponents insert subjective values into the process that bias their results toward a higher ratio. Discount rates are used to convert expected future benefits and costs into current value. Some argue that this allows proponents of a project to undervalue the impact on future generations, for instance, with regard to potential economic impacts of global climate change.

Uncertainty can be included in BCA by allowing confidence limit bands to increase over time. However, this step can provide opportunities for project insiders to manipulate the outcomes. One of the most persistent criticisms of BCA is that it puts a monetary value on human life and environmental assets, even if economic values come from court decisions. It is fair to say that, in general, economists and business interests favor BCA. The flip side is that many others do not. Some are distressed by efforts to express all impacts as monetary outcomes, which they consider to be a perversion of the belief that quality of life is what is most important.

We believe that strong feelings about BCA are partly attributable to its long history. The idea of comparing the benefits and costs is attributable to Jules Dupuit, a French engineer, who wrote on the topic more than 150 years ago.[28] BCA began to have a substantial influence on decisions made by the U.S. government after floods struck and killed thousands and destroyed multiple communities during the 1930s. The Flood Control Act of 1939 sought to protect people and property, and choices had to be made among proposed projects. BCA was required as a tool to guide decision-makers.

The impacts of BCA were at first positive because disastrous flooding had to be managed. Indeed, flood control has been identified as the second major environmental management program in the United States (the third, pollution control, led to NEPA and the EIS process).[29] As flood control projects continued, however, BCA was blamed for some unpopular decisions. The epitome of the criticism was a book by Heuvelmans, *The River Killers*.[30] The cover of this book showed a dagger stabbed into a river, indicating that flood control projects have far exceeded their need.

During the past 80 years, BCA has been extended to land conservation, recreation, water quantity and quality, college education, and many other policy issues. In fact, BCA became a major tool under President Ronald Reagan, who wanted all federal policies to be valued for costs and benefits. Reagan created the Office of Information and Regulatory Affairs (OIRA), charging it with reviewing regulations that were expected to cost more than $100 million a year. It goes without saying that BCA carries controversy with it to whatever policy area to which it is applied. Yet OIRA's work continues to contribute to the decision-making process, despite efforts by some to persuade every president, both Democrat and Republican, to eliminate or curtail its powers.

Notwithstanding the criticism of BCA, it is not inertia that keeps this tool viable as a decision-making aid. It fills a need for more detailed information about the size of benefits and costs (and winners and losers) in the decision-making process. It fills the role that the EIS plays in environmental policy and that risk analysis plays in complex risk-related projects. Like these other tools, those in authority are going to use some form of BCA to better understand the implications of their decisions. Federal agencies such as the Federal Aviation Administration, Federal Highway Administration, and the Transportation Research Board provide guidance, and software packages are widely available for performing BCA with varying levels of complexity.[25,31]

Some alternatives to BCA are available for specific applications. One of these is cost–effectiveness analysis, which compares the costs and outcomes of multiple options for addressing an issue. For example, what kind of investments should government make to encourage the goal of reducing fossil fuel use?[27] Each option can be evaluated without as many assumptions as are required in BCA.

In the case of local-scale projects, many communities use fiscal impact analysis. This method calculates economic costs and benefits of new land uses, including contributing inexpensive land, tax credits, and other benefits.[32] In regard to health care benefits and costs, some prefer cost–utility analysis,[33] which includes many of the ideas of cost–effectiveness analysis and estimates costs relative to the expected health outcomes measured both in quality and quantity of life.

Case Study: Denver International Airport

After more than three hours of traveling, seeing the Rocky Mountains while descending into DIA from the East Coast was a welcome relief. The airport is massive, the people movers are easy to navigate, the airport terminals look like teepees, and the airport is filled with interesting art. Before 1996, landing in Denver, Colorado, was not nearly as memorable. Stapleton Airport, built in 1929, was functional, but it was neither attractive nor well located. It was like other airports where the facilities are squeezed for space and not much can be done to add additional runways or expand terminals. One advantage of Stapleton was that it only took 18 to 20 minutes to get from Stapleton to downtown Denver.

With the expectation that the Denver region would grow and that Denver was a logical hub for tourists and businesses, the City of Denver and the County of Denver proposed abandoning Stapleton and building a new airport east of the Rocky Mountain Arsenal. Most of the land was part of Adams County, which required a referendum that a substantial majority of voters approved in 1988.[34]

The DIA considered in the FEIS[35] was built 25 miles from downtown Denver, and it takes about 35 minutes to get to the Colorado Convention Center by car in light traffic (Figure 9.1). A great deal of political and social networking was part of this process, which continues. This case study, however, does not focus on these tools. Rather, it focuses on the use of the EIS process in decision-making, the regional economic impact of the airport, and the use of BCE as part of the case for airport expansion.

The search for a new airport location began with the assumption that it would be located north and east of the mountains west of Denver and away from the city and other existing population centers. The Federal Aviation Administration (FAA) was the lead agency for the EIS process, and the Federal Highway Administration was a cooperating agency because of the need to link the airport with the developed and developing parts of the region. As is the norm for a large EIS, the city and county of Denver designated personnel to work on the EIS. However, a good deal of the work was done by consultants who provided information to the designated personnel and received feedback from them on technical issues. Technical issues included information on air traffic management, terminal design, lighting, and many others, as well as many environmental management issues.

Following standard protocols, 19 representatives of federal, state, and local agencies listened and spoke at the initial meetings. They were all encouraged to submit written comments and 11 of them did. Four public meetings were held to solicit input. The major issues raised at the meetings were noise, land use and development, air quality, automobile traffic and interchanges, revitalization of the Stapleton airport area, and impact on local schools in nearby Aurora.

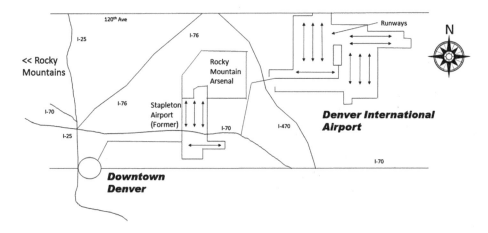

Note: Locations are not to scale in order to emphasize key sites, and selected routes are shown. Travel time to downtown Denver from Denver International Airport by automobile is 30 to 40 minutes.

Figure 9.1. Location Sketch of Denver International Airport

The DEIS was circulated and parties were provided with time to respond, albeit there are always requests for additional time. As is the norm, letters from the public were received, made part of the record, and addressed by the technical staff.

EISs have a no-action alternative and one or more other options. They almost always have a preferred one. In this case, the no-action alternative was keeping Stapleton open and the other alternatives were various numbers of runways and directions built east and north of Denver.

After receiving input, the EIS research team focused on the following issues:

- Noise
- Land use
- Social impacts
- Surface transportation
- Induced socioeconomic impacts
- Air quality
- Water quality
- Department of Transportation Act section 4(f) (land in the vicinity of an airport)
- Historical/archaeological
- Biotic communities
- Endangered species
- Wetlands
- Floodplains and hydrology
- Coastal zone management, coastal barriers, and wild and scenic rivers

- Farmlands
- Energy supply and natural resources
- Solid waste impact
- Light emissions
- Construction impacts
- Design, art
- Mitigation actions

Although each of these issues was considered in the FEIS,[35] we focus next on several that appear to have been the most critical.

Noise

Noise attracted a great deal of attention. The FAA has an integrated noise model that calculates a cumulative noise exposure metric. Loudness day night (Ldn) means a decibel noise level that will not produce distressed residents, which the FAA sets at 65 Ldn.[35] The FAA noise model draws sound contours around approaches and runways. It is important to know that decibel is a logarithmic scale, which means that a 10-decibel increase means an increase in power by a factor of 10. Hence, an increase from 60 to 70 decibels represents a massive increase in power impacting the ear (see Table 5.1 for two checklist questions that assess day and night decibel levels that typically lead to public protests).

The no-action alternative, continuing to use Stapleton, produced much higher public exposure numbers to noise than any of the alternatives that use the proposed site (Table 9.2).

The FEIS provided multiple noise contour diagrams that assume different runway configurations and uses at various times. In short, the new Denver airport would substantially reduce the number of people in the 65 Ldn or higher zone.

Table 9.2. Public Exposure to Noise Estimates for Alternatives to the Denver International Airport

Alternative	Population Exposed, Ldn 65
At time of EIS	14,666
No-action alternative, 1995	14,389
No-action alternative, 2020[a]	1,238
New airport: Phase 1	518 to 559
New airport completed	388 to 410

Source: Based on U.S. Department of Transportation (1989).[35(p.vii–ix)]
Note: EIS = environmental impact statement; Ldn = loudness day night.
[a]Assumes acquisition of less noisy aircraft at Stapleton by 2020.

Table 9.3. Forecast for Airport Use in the Denver Area

Year	Passenger Enplanements[a]	Volume of Air Carrier
1975	6,411	211
1980	9,789	317
1985	14,387	339
1990 forecast	18,789	392
1995 forecast[b]	26,500 to 28,000	552 to 600
2000 forecast[b]	32,000 to 34,000	600 to 700

Source: Based on U.S. Department of Transportation (1989).[35(p1-2)]
[a]Avoids double-counting people by counting people that board.
[b]Assumes a new airport.

Regional Socioeconomic Impacts

The FEIS and supporting documents assumed substantial growth in the use of airports. Table 9.3 lists the forecast for use of the airport in Denver as presented in the FEIS.

A concern expressed in the FEIS is that Denver would lose its existing position as a hub for several airlines if a new airport with longer runways was not available. Specifically, Stapleton had six runways, but they were not long enough or spaced far enough apart to provide maximum flexibility for air traffic. Weather conditions can change quickly in the Denver area, and the runway lengths and configurations limited the capacity for takeoffs and landing, leading to delays. The FEIS argued that these delays are then propagated across the entire nation. Using 1987 data, the FEIS reported that Stapleton was one of the five most constrained domestic U.S. airports. It estimated that a new Denver airport would reduce delays 4.8 percent nationally, a reduction of about 200 hours daily delay across the nation.

The FEIS was approved by the FAA, and the airport opened in 1996. The new airport encompassed 33,531 acres (52.4 square miles, or 135.7 square kilometers), making it the largest airport in the United States. Five of its six runways were 12,000 feet long, allowing the airport to keep up with the requirements of new and larger aircraft for takeoffs and landings.

The FAA is one of the major users of BCA.[25] To build a sixth runway, DIA's management had to demonstrate that adding a new runway would make the airport more efficient. Consultants used FAA BCA models to estimate the benefits, finding that adding a sixth runway (north–south) would reduce, on average, 0.9 minutes from each aircraft takeoff and landing. This was applied to flights and yielded an annual average of $9.6 million in benefit to the airlines, and $2.1 million in passenger time savings.[36,37] The cost of the runway was estimated at $154.7 million, of which DIA asked the federal government for up to $120 million. The runway was added, which is 16,000 feet long

(4,877 meters and longest commercial runway in the United States) for new heavy jumbo jets. Although the cost sounds enormous, the runway was actually cheap compared with other airports because the DIA already owned the land. By contrast, adding a runway to Chicago, Illinois; San Francisco, California; and New York City–northern New Jersey airports might be cost-prohibitive because these airports are adjacent to existing urban land uses. These airports would have to purchase occupied land or build a new runway over existing bodies of water.

The DIA cost and benefit report estimated a total benefit of $731 million in savings over a 20-year period, a very good benefit-to-cost ratio. In 2000, DIA released a report that they had begun building the new 16,000 foot runway that would allow them to land planes during harsh conditions on the existing north–south runways and use the new runway for takeoffs. In their press release, DIA reported a cost of "only" $166 million and cited a savings to the national aviation system of more than $1 billion over the life of the runway, a benefit-to-cost ratio of 12 to 1.[38]

A key argument for building the airport was that Stapleton could not handle the air traffic that a new airport could and that Stapleton was destined for very long flight delays. Recent U.S. Department of Transportation data show that even the new DIA airport has among the lowest rates of on-time departures. Among the 29 most used airports in 2012 and 2013, DIA ranked 28th and 26th, respectively.[39] These results are not subtle. Airports with more flights (75,000+) had far fewer flight delays than those with far fewer flights. For example, the 10 U.S. airports with fewer than 1,000 flights ranked 1 through 7, 9, 11, and 13 in regard to on-time departures. Those with more than 75,000 flights ranked between 113 and 295. Denver ranked 272, a little worse than many of its large counterparts. In other words, even the large new DIA cannot easily cope with the increasing demands and the vagaries of the weather.[40] Flying into Stapleton with the amount of traffic that DIA has would be a major assault on a passenger's patience and blood pressure.

Although DIA is not among the best with regard to on-time take-offs, it certainly has expanded its service. The airport is the main hub for Frontier and Great Lakes airlines. Other major users include United and Southwest. The airport, according to DIA, has enough space to add more runways and accommodate up to 110 million passengers, up from 32 million in 1996 and 54 million in 2015 when it ranked fifth in passenger traffic.[41,42]

The FEIS did not use any of the regional economic impact models described earlier in this chapter. Nevertheless, at the regional scale, the FEIS points to airport, land use, and road transportation changes that would add 4,100 hotel rooms, 425,000 square feet of air cargo and freight forwarding space, and an additional 150,000 square feet of office space, car rental and airport services space.[35]

The Colorado Department of Transportation used an I–O model to estimate the economic impact of all of Colorado's airports, of which DIA is by far the largest.[41,43] The DIA's

Table 9.4. Percentage of Impacts Generated On and Off Site at the Denver International Airport

Economic Category	On-Site Impacts	Off-Site Multiplier Impacts
Jobs	59%	41%
Payroll $	58%	42%
Output	57%	43%

Source: Based on data from Colorado Department of Transportation (2013).[41]

estimated economic impact was $26.3 billion in 2013; the airport was responsible for 188,000 jobs. Specifically, the airport's on-site impacts were attributed to administration, airport tenants, and capital investment. Off-site impacts included spending by commercial visitors, general aviation visitors, and businesses using air cargo. There were also tax revenues from retail sales, lodging, food and beverages, entertainment, recreation, local transportation, rental cars, and construction.

The initial impacts and the multiplier effects from the State of Colorado's I–O model results are shown in Table 9.4.

The table shows that almost 60 percent of the airport's economic impact is estimated to be generated on site, with the remaining 40 percent off site. Suffice it to say that not all of DIA's investments have been successful. The automated baggage moving system failed and had to be abandoned. The initial estimated cost of the airport was $2.8 billion, whereas the final cost was $4.8 billion and the opening was delayed by 16 months. Yet, on the positive side of the ledger, DIA not only has beautiful terminals but also spacious ones that contain wonderful art. Notably, the DIA was the first U.S. airport to be certified by ISO-14001[44] for environmental management, a status that is based on a full range of environmental issues relevant to its operations. These include sewer and water systems, air emissions, waste management, climate change mitigation, and use of resources and water. The DIA has multiple solar fields, Wi-Fi access throughout the airport, and it takes about 35 to 40 minutes to travel from downtown Denver by a rail system built specifically for the airport.

Stapleton Airport Redevelopment

One of the public concerns in the FEIS is what would happen to the old Stapleton Airport area. The FEIS calls for closing and rehabilitating Stapleton airport, which was expected to reduce automobile traffic in the Stapleton area. The FEIS indicates that 6,400 dwelling units were likely to be built on the old Stapleton airport site by the year 2020, along with workplaces, schools, a regional shopping center, and other facilities.[35]

Indeed, a new urban settlement has been constructed on the 7.35 square mile site (19 square kilometers). The area includes more than 3,000 single-family homes, condominiums, and row houses; 400 apartments; and multiple commercial enterprises and parks. Located about 15 miles from downtown Denver, the Stapleton area is served by a rail line and expects to be home to 30,000 people. The design of the new settlement is consistent with the New Urbanism (see Chapters 2 and 11 on this topic), sporting a great deal of diversity in housing options and multiple amenities, which are advertised on the Stapleton Web site.[45]

A decade after the new Stapleton community opened, Raabe[46] assessed the new development as having growing pains. With 15,000 to 20,000 residents, he notes that the $5 billion investment has been praised and won awards from the U.S. Conference of Mayors, the Urban Land Institute, the National League of Cities, and the EPA for building sustainability concepts into its plans. However, Raabe also notes that some residents are concerned about the lack of retailing in general and walkable shopping more specifically. There is also less open space than expected. Some residents voiced concern at the abandonment of office space in favor of residential development. One expert observed that the Stapleton plan is among the most complex of urban redevelopment projects and expectations are so high that perfection is not possible. The EIS's population expectations will probably fall a bit short by 2020, but not by much.

Considering the number of EISs we have read, the FEIS for the DIA is relatively easy to follow and seems to have forecasted a good deal of what has happened. Of course, a good EIS should be a good blueprint for what actually happens on the ground.

Case Study: Liquefied Natural Gas—Economic Impact Models in a Changing Economy

This case study highlights the unquestionable bottom-line importance of the profit motive in decision-making. It focuses on the need to address not only impacts that frighten people but also those that are likely to be challenging to manage. It also addresses the need to be skeptical about models and the assumptions built into models, especially those that are not transparent and publicly available.

Sparrows Point Application

LNG is natural gas that is cooled to less than −260° Fahrenheit (−161° Celsius). At that temperature, the gas is compressed to one-600th of its natural volume, which means that it can be economically transported long distances in large ships. In 2006, the AES Corporation, a large energy company with power plants and utilities in more than 20 countries and 25,000 employees, proposed to build an LNG plant at a former steel mill site at Sparrows

Table 9.5. Impacts Considered in the Sparrows Point Environmental Impact Statement

Impact[a]	
Air Quality and Noise • Air quality • Noise	**Soils** • LNG terminal site • Waterway
Cultural Resources • Results of cultural resource surveys • Native Americans • Unanticipated discoveries • Compliance with the NHPA (Section 106)	**Terrestrial and Aquatic Species** • Terrestrial species • Aquatic species • Essential fish habitat
Geological Resources • Physiologic and geologic setting • Other natural hazards • Paleontological natural hazards	**Threatened, Endangered, and Other Special-Status Species** • Federally listed threatened and endangered species • Federally listed species on the marine transit route • State-listed threatened and endangered species and other species of concern
Land-Use, Recreation, and Visual Resources • Land use • Existing and planned residences and developments • Coastal zone management • Hazardous waste sites • Recreation and public interest areas • Visual resources	**Water Resources** • Groundwater • Surface water
Reliability and Safety • LNG hazard • Front-end engineering design and review • Storage and retention systems • Siting requirements • LNG vessel safety • Emergency response and evaluation planning • Conclusions on LNG vessel safety • Terrorism and security issues • Pipeline safety standards • Pipeline accident data • Impact on public safety	**Wetlands** • Regulatory permits • Wetland types impacted by the proposed project • Potential impacts of the Mid-Atlantic Express Pipeline to wetlands • Wetlands construction and maintenance procedures and aquatic resources mitigation plan
Socioeconomics • Population, economy, and employment • Housing • Public services • Transportation and vehicle traffic • Property values • Environmental justice	**Vegetation** • Vegetation resources • Vegetation management plan • Noxious weeds • Vegetation monitoring conclusions

Source: Based on Greenberg 2012[10] and Federal Energy and Regulatory Commission 2008.[47]
Note: LNG = liquefied natural gas; NHPA = National Historic Preservation Act.
[a]Impacts are cumulative.

Point, Maryland. Sparrows Point is located on a small peninsula in Baltimore County, just southeast of the City of Baltimore, about 17 miles from the inner harbor area.

Table 9.5 lists the major environmental impacts and their subcategories included in the Sparrows Point EIS. This EIS is typical insofar as it does cover every one of these categories without fail. Some are more important than others; however, each had to be considered in order to avoid court challenges based on neglect of a key potential impact. Here we focus on several issues that drew a lot of public attention and some others that drew much less but were at least as important.

LNG can catch on fire and some argued that it could explode. These health and safety concerns were emphasized both at the public hearings and through the mail. Nevertheless, technical experts persuaded federal agencies that there would be no explosion and a serious fire was highly unlikely. Not everyone was persuaded, including the Fire Chief of the adjacent community (Dundalk) who argued that if a fire occurred, it could not be put out because of the extremely high temperature. This fear never dissipated and experts could not deny that there have been fires, including several at LNG facilities in the United States, but not in the recent past.[10,47]

Tanker collisions were a second major concern. New LNG tankers are more than 1,100 feet (345 meters) long and more than 145 feet (45 meters) wide, with striking ball-shape tanks visible from above (see Figure 9.2). These tankers are about the size of a modern day aircraft carrier and, even though they are required to have two hulls, the U.S. Coast Guard challenged their ability to be safely operated in the region and noted concern about collisions. The public was told that the tankers would be accompanied by tugboats during the 165-mile trip up Chesapeake Bay to Sparrows Point, that notice of their schedule would be provided, and that other ships would not be permitted in the area during that period of time. Nevertheless, many members of the community did not accept these explanations as adequate.

Dredging the channel so that the large tankers could navigate the Chesapeake was less of a focal point than was the potential for explosions, fires, and collisions, which truly disturbed the local population. Local environmental and planning officials brought up the issue of dredging as the Sparrows Point EIS estimated that 3,700,000 cubic yards of material would have to be dredged.[47] Dredging stirs up sediments, including toxins; however, this issue was not a prominent discussion point in the EIS process. Dredge materials must also be transported to another site. AES estimated that 220 truck trips a day would be required to haul the dredged material. We cannot imagine that this would not have been a major issue for local transportation planners and public health officials, given the reality that dredge spills do occur, along with their associated noxious odors and unsightly appearance. The ideas of using dredge materials to cap landfills, placing them in abandoned mines, and using them for other purposes were noted in the FEIS. Although these ideas are feasible, insufficient details about the options were provided in the document.

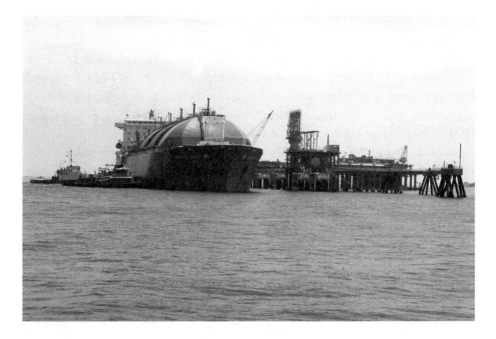

Source: Reprinted from U.S. Coast Guard.[48]
Note: Consider the vessel's size.

Figure 9.2. Liquefied Natural Gas Tanker

In the end, this FEIS is not among the strongest that we have read. There was a notable lack of socioeconomic impact analysis, a limited analysis of the long-term need for LNG in the region, and a lack of a satisfactory environmental justice presentation. Nevertheless, it is also fair to say that, without the EIS process, and the slow painstaking work done to prepare and review the EIS, this roughly $1 billion terminal and pipeline extensions would have been built.

What actually happened was what we would characterize as "death by 1,000 cuts." The State of Maryland's political leadership and the local communities wanted the proposal to be rejected. The applicant had to satisfy many conditions to receive approval, which took an enormous amount of time and cost a great deal of money. In the end, the company stopped the process, not the government or the opponents.

The Sparrows Point EIS process illustrates not only the siting of a prominent kind of locally unwanted land use but also how difficult preparing an EIS can be for the applicant and those challenging a major economic environment project. This case study also illustrates a regulatory EIS. Indeed, EISs prepared by regulatory agencies typically lead to conditional "yes" decisions whereby the applicant can build as long as they satisfy many conditions. In this case, construction practices, operations, mitigation resources, Coast Guard approvals, security measures, and many others placed roadblocks in the way of this project. There were 169 conditions attached to an approval of the application by the federal agencies.

AES withdrew its application to build an LNG facility at Sparrows Point in 2013 without explanation.[49] One possible reason is the strong opposition they faced. Another is that the company never received a permit to dredge the area around the proposed site, which was required for the large tankers. We speculate that the most compelling reason for AES having dropped their application is that the natural gas market markedly changed between 2006 and 2013. Gas prices fell because of domestic and oil shale production, and AES no longer saw the local market for LNG that it had anticipated. Instead of importing LNG from Nigeria, Trinidad, Indonesia, Qatar, and other places, the United States became an exporter. Domestic prices were half of what had been expected by the company and the need for a project to import LNG essentially evaporated.

The United States as a Liquefied Natural Gas Exporter

The Sparrows Point LNG case study began with the premise that the United States needed to import natural gas for domestic distribution, but it ends in a very different place. U.S. gas production increased 20 percent between 2005 and 2009. While domestic natural gas prices plunged, other countries such as Japan (which lost and shut down its nuclear power plants) and China (with its vastly expanding economy) needed more energy. With the availability of shale gas obtained through fracking, the United States became an exporting nation. Although the United States has obligations to its trade partners, it does not have obligations to ship LNG to China, India, or Japan.[50,51]

An interesting "battle of the printouts" resulting from complex economic models addressing U.S. exports of LNG began in August 2011. That is when the Office of Fossil Energy within the U.S. Department of Energy requested that the Energy Information Administration (EIA) conduct a study to understand how U.S. exports of LNG would impact the nation—in particular, the energy and manufacturing sectors.[51] Federal laws require the United States to export natural gas to countries with which it has trade agreements, but not necessarily to those without a trade agreement. Hence, the federal government needed some idea of how increasing LNG shipments would impact the environment, energy security, and the nation's economy.

The EIA asked consultants to address four scenarios for increased exports in natural gas[44]:

1. Slow: 6 billion cubic feet per day (Bcf/d) phased in at a rate of 1 Bcf/d per year
2. Low–rapid: 6 Bcf/d phased in at 3 Bcf/d per year
3. High–slow: 12 Bcf/d phased in at a rate of 1 Bcf/d per year
4. High–rapid: 12 Bcf/d phased in at a rate of 3 Bcf/day per year

The report noted that Canada and Mexico already receive natural gas via pipeline and have a free-trade agreement with the United States. It mentioned that South Korea is a major possible client for LNG, but only if that country also signs a free-trade agreement. The report noted that existing economic models are not able to capture worldwide impacts because global gas markets are not integrated and wide fluctuations in prices and sales of LNG can occur. As a result, investments in LNG plants are expensive whereas the payoff for these investments is uncertain. It is also possible that countries such as Nigeria or Venezuela might be able to build less costly LNG plants, but they have politically volatile environments.[44]

The authors of this book have used and built regional economic impact models, and the LNG case illustrates why we use the following six questions when considering the results produced by complex models:

1. What kind of model(s) is being used? Is the description clear? Can you trace it back to the literature? What does the literature say are strengths and weaknesses of this type of model?
2. What kind of data and assumptions are input into the model? Have the assumptions been made clear? Are the data publicly available, and can you find them?
3. Is the model proprietary? Is it a model that only the analyst can understand and use?
4. Does that model produce geographical results? At what scales?
5. Does the model produce time series results? For what time periods?
6. What have analysts written about this type of model and this specific model?

NERA, an economic consulting firm, used its economic models to study the relationship between export levels and domestic prices. They have a global natural gas model[52] and a macroeconomic model,[53] which are described as having the capacity to "forecast the impact of policy, regulatory, and economic factors on the energy sectors and the economy."[53(p20)] With minor adjustments to account for the U.S. recovery from the early 21st century recession and differential impacts on economic sectors, the results from its 2012 and 2014 reports are not significantly altered.[54] They are that

• Macroeconomic impacts of LNG exports are positive to the U.S. economy in every scenario.
• Unlimited exports produce the most benefits.
• LNG export potential is greater because gas prices dropped.
• U.S. manufacturing rebirth would unlikely to be harmed by LNG exports.
• LNG exports would hasten return to full employment.

These simple conclusions belie the complexity of the economic modeling NERA did and the underlying assumptions embedded in their studies. The appendices detailing the model provide enough information to tell us what they did, but not enough detail to know precisely how they did it. The report includes some explanations about the assumptions, but not many. We learn that NERA used several models to estimate impacts at the national scale. The base of the model is the year 2008 IMPLAN I–O model of 440 different economic sectors. The results are projected forward with the most recent U.S. government forecasts, using optimization models to drive the economy toward an equilibrium state. In other words, the model is far from transparent.

The EIA called for comments on the NERA report. Synapse, an energy economics consulting group with a portfolio of energy sustainability environmental projects, provided a detailed critique. The group reported that[52,53]

- With the exception of the gas industry, the proposed project would lead to a decline in U.S. gross domestic product.
- Major job losses would occur, which are not calculated by the Montgomery and Tuladhar report,[53] and Synapse estimated that between 36,000 and 270,000 jobs would be lost per year with a median of 131,000.
- Potential severe impacts on some businesses and population are ignored.
- Wage earners in every sector, except natural gas, lose income.
- Impacts on electricity prices are not calculated by the Montgomery and Tuladhar study[53] and should have been.
- The assertion of widespread stock ownership benefits is not supported; only the most affluent would benefit.
- The claim that some of the international benefits of exports will return to U.S. residents is not supported by historical studies that show many of the benefits will remain overseas.
- The assumption that anyone who wants a job can get one is unrealistic, as is the assumption that monetary policy will not change.

The Synapse critique of the NERA report is not surprising. The problem is that the NERA models are not available to be scrutinized and the results are aspatial (without geographic definition). The NERA report also lacks an environmental impact discussion. Without access to the models, we cannot say if we would have arrived at the same sweeping policy conclusions as either NERA or Synapse. It is also painful to see a set of macroeconomic results on a subject like this that does not separate the results for the Great Lakes and Northeast from the Southwest and Alaska (see also other LNG studies[55,56]).

When this chapter was written, we had seen only one study on LNG that provides sufficient regional and time series data to make the results useful to local planners and health officials. Treyz et al. began to address these shortcomings by combining elements of I–O analysis, econometrics, CGE, and REMI to produce an exceedingly complicated analysis of the LNG export issue.[57] The results were estimated for each of the 50 states and Washington, D.C. The models included 169 industrial sectors, which closely correspond with the classification that the U.S. government uses to gather business data. The models were combined with a natural gas market model that estimates flows of natural gas based on demand and prices, which is consistent with what gas traders actually do.

The Treyz et al. models are complex, and we cannot do justice to them here. They clearly show, however, that results vary not only by how much is exported but also by place and time. For example, the higher the exports, the more the impacts. This is especially true at first because facilities are constructed to facilitate the exports. Texas, Louisiana, Alaska, and Dominion Cove Point, Maryland, are places with existing facilities and capacities that are likely to be the major beneficiaries. By contrast, the Midwest manufacturing belt in Ohio, Michigan, Illinois, and elsewhere around the Great Lakes suffers losses because they use a great deal of gas and would face higher prices because of exports. If you live in any of these areas, local benefits and costs from global market changes are absolutely critical to helping you understand what would happen to your tax revenues, income, and the potential for population changes in the area, along with resources for schools and public health.

The LNG story continues to unfold. In May 2014, the *Economist*[58] reported that the international market for LNG was growing and would rise more than 70 percent between 2014 and 2020. The author of the article wonders how large a part the United States is willing to play in supplying these resources. The facilities in Texas, Louisiana, and Maryland have already begun shipping LNG, but other countries such as Qatar, Australia, and Russia can ship LNG to the Far East at a lower price. The LNG market is too unstable to know with any confidence how much U.S. companies should invest and how much support the federal government should provide. What is clear is that increased investments in select economic sectors will doubtless provoke some negative environmental consequences and strong public perceptions.

Overall, it is hard to take the results from limited economic models (the battle of the printouts) at face value because they ignore environmental and human health and safety, are proprietary, and are inscrutable even to those who understand the tools. The results pose a dilemma for decision-makers and for public health and planners who have been handed complex results from black box tools that they cannot open or question. Nevertheless, readers of this book would be well served to understand the basics of the models in order to ask informed questions that may yield important insights about the underlying assumptions. We recommend you review the six questions presented earlier as a start in that direction.

Final Thoughts

You may not trust the EIS process, the qualitative judgments in BCA, or the underlying assumptions and complexity of economic modeling, yet these tools cannot be ignored because they are required by legal mandates and have been part of federal decision-making for decades. The EIS process is far from a rubber stamp. It has caused proposals to be canceled and many to be markedly modified. BCA is required for many public and privately supported projects. Regional economic impact models are imperfect, but they provide clues about where and when impacts will occur, as well as their magnitude. The public health and planning practitioner who is not familiar with these three tools will not have a firm basis to object to or support the findings and conclusions drawn from their results. Without the capacity to understand and ask questions about those results, you will find it difficult to confront boosterism and NIMBYism. Unfortunately, back-of-the-envelope calculations will not work for projects of the scale described in this chapter.

References

1. Seley JD. *Politics of Public-Facility Planning*. Lexington, MA: Rowman and Littlefield; 1983.

2. O'Hare M. *Facility Siting and Public Opposition*. New York, NY: Van Nostrand Reinhold; 1983.

3. Boholm A, Löfstedt R. *Facility Siting: Risk, Power and Identity in Land Use Planning*. Sterling, VA: Earthscan; 2004.

4. Portney KE. *Siting Hazardous Waste Treatment Facilities: The NIMBY Syndrome*. New York, NY: Praeger; 1991.

5. Lindell M, Earle T. How close is close enough: public perceptions of the risks of industrial facilities. *Risk Anal.* 1983;3:245–253.

6. Greenberg MR, Popper FJ, Truelove HB. Are LULUs still enduringly objectionable? *J Environ Plan Manag.* 2012;55(6):713–731.

7. Congressional Declaration of National Environmental Policy, Title 1, Sec. 101, 42 USC §4331 (1970):1.

8. US Congress. National Environmental Policy Act of 1969 (As Amended). Available at: https://energy.gov/sites/prod/files/nepapub/nepa_documents/RedDont/Req-NEPA.pdf Accessed September 3, 2016.

9. Council on Environmental Quality. A Citizen's Guide to the NEPA: Having Your Voice Heard. Executive Office of the President. 2007. Available at: https://energy.gov/nepa/downloads/citizens-guide-nepa-having-your-voice-heard-ceq-2007. Accessed March 11, 2017.

10. Greenberg MR. *The Environmental Impact Statement After Two Generations: Managing Environmental Power*. New York, NY: Routledge; 2012.

11. Greenberg M, Anderson R, Page G. *Environmental Impact Statements*. Resource Papers for College Geography 78–83, Washington, DC: Association of American Geographers; 1978.

12. State of California. California Environmental Quality Act. 2014. Available at: http://resources.ca.gov/ceqa/more/faq.html#guidelines. Accessed March 11, 2017.

13. City and County of San Francisco Planning Department. Environmental review process. Available at: http://sf-planning.org/environmental-review-process. Accessed September 3, 2016.

14. US Government Accountability Office. National Environmental Policy Act: Little information exists on NEPA analyses. GAO-14-369. 2014. Available at: http://www.gao.gov/products/GAO-14-370. Accessed September 3, 2016.

15. Greenberg MR, Lahr M, Mantell N. Understanding the economic costs and benefits of catastrophes and their aftermath: a review and suggestions for the US Federal Government. *Risk Anal.* 2007;27(1):83–96.

16. Hill R, Griffiths W, Lim G. *Principles of Econometrics.* 4th ed. New York, NY: John Wiley & Sons; 2011.

17. Judge G, Hill R, Griffiths W, Lutkepohl H, Lee T. *Introduction to the Theory and Practice of Econometrics.* New York, NY: John Wiley & Sons; 1982.

18. Miller R, Blair P. *Input–Output Analysis: Foundations and Extensions.* New York, NY: Cambridge University Press; 2009.

19. Partridge M, Rickman D. Regional computable general equilibrium modeling: a survey and critical appraisal. *Int Reg Sci.* 1998;21(3):205–248.

20. Rose A, Liao S-Y. Modeling regional economic resilience to disasters: a computable general equilibrium analysis of water service disruptions. *J Reg Sci.* 2005;45(1):75–112.

21. Treyz G. *Regional Economic Modeling: A Systematic Approach to Economic Forecasting and Policy Analysis.* Boston, MA: Kluwer Academic Publishers; 1993.

22. The REMI EDFS-53 Forecasting & Simulation Model, Volume 1, Model Documentation. Amherst, MA: REMI Inc; 1997.

23. Pearce DW, Atkinson G, Mourato S. Cost-benefit analysis and the environment: recent developments. Paris, France: Organisation for Economic Co-operation and Development; 2006.

24. Pearce D. Cost benefit analysis and environmental policy. *Oxford Rev Econ Policy.* 1998;14(4):84–100.

25. *FAA Airport Benefit–Cost Analysis Guidance.* Washington, DC: Office of Aviation Policy and Plans; 1999.

26. Mishan EJ, Quah E. *Cost–Benefit Analysis.* 5th ed. New York, NY: Routledge; 2007.

27. Levin H, McEwan P. *Cost-Effectiveness Analysis: Methods and Applications.* Thousand Oaks, CA: Sage Publications; 2001.

28. Ekelund R. Jules Dupuit and the early theory of marginal cost pricing. *J Polit Econ.* 1968;76(3):462–471.

29. Dunlap RE, Mertig AG. The evolution of the US environmental movement from 1970 to 1990: an overview. *Soc Nat Resour.* 1991;4(3):209–218.

30. Heuvelmans M. *The River Killers.* Mechanicsburg, PA: Stackpole Books; 1974.

31. Director of Civil Works' Policy Memorandum CWPM 12-001. Methodology for Updating Benefit-to-Cost Ratios (BCR) for Budget Development. Washington, DC: US Army Corps of Engineers; 2012.

32. Burchell R, Listokin D. *The Fiscal Impact Handbook: Estimating Local Costs and Revenues of Land Development.* New Brunswick, NJ: Center for Urban Policy Research/Transaction Press; 1978.

33. Cheng AK, Rubin HR, Powe NR, et al. Cost–utility analysis of the cochlear implant in children. *JAMA.* 2000;284(7):850–856.

34. Weiner E. Voters in Denver approve a new $2.3 billion airport. *New York Times.* May 16, 1989. Available at: http://www.nytimes.com/1989/05/17/us/voters-in-denver-approve-a-new-2.3-billion-airport.html. Accessed March 11, 2017.

35. US Department of Transportation, Federal Aviation Administration. *Final Environmental Impact Statement, New Denver Airport, volume 1.* 1989. Available at: http://www.flydenver.com/sites/default/files/environmental/finalEIS1989.pdf. Accessed September 4, 2016.

36. Denver International Airport. Managing the environment at Denver International Airport. 2011. Available at: http://www.flydenver.com/about/administration/environmental_management. Accessed September 4, 2016.

37. Leib J. DIA weighs 6th runway to save time. *The Denver Post.* April 20, 2000: Business News. Available at: http://extras.denverpost.com/business/biz0420c.htm. Accessed September 4, 2016.

38. Denver International Airport. Paving begins on Denver International Airport's sixth runway. May 2002. Available at: https://www.flydenver.com/sites/default/files/downloads/DIAPR_020606_1.pdf. Accessed March 11, 2017.

39. Travelmath. 2015 Travelmath.com airport rankings. 2015. Available at: http://www.travelmath.com/feature/airport-rankings. Accessed September 4, 2016.

40. US Department of Transportation, Bureau of Transportation Statistics. Ranking of major airport on-time departure performance in February 2013. Available at: https://www.rita.dot.gov/bts/subject_areas/airline_information/airline_ontime_tables/2013_02/table_05. Accessed August 8, 2017.

41. Colorado Department of Transportation. *2013 Economic Impact Study of Colorado Airports.* Available at: https://www.codot.gov/programs/aeronautics/Economic Impact Study. Accessed September 4, 2016.

42. Wikipedia. Denver International Airport. 2016. Available at: https://en.wikipedia.org/wiki/Denver_International_Airport. Accessed March 11, 2017.

43. MIG, formerly Minnesota IMPLAN Group I. Economic impact modeling. 2016. Available at: http://implan.com. Accessed September 4, 2016.

44. International Standards Organzation. ISO 14001:2015 Environmental management systems. 2015. Available at: http://www.iso.org/iso/home/store/catalogue_tc/catalogue_detail.htm?csnumber=60857. Accessed September 4, 2016.

45. Stapleton Denver. Home. 2016. Available at: http://www.stapletondenver.com. Accessed September 4, 2016.

46. Raabe S. As Stapleton neighborhood prepares to expand north, residents want south projects finished. *Denver Post*. February 17, 2012. Available at: http://www.denverpost. com/2012/02/17/as-stapleton-neighborhood-prepares-to-expand-north-residents-want-south-projects-finished. Accessed March 11, 2017.

47. *Sparrows Point LNG and Mid-Atlantic Express Pipeline Project DEIS*. Washington, DC; Federal Energy and Regulatory Commission; 2008.

48. US Coast Guard. Liquefied natural gas tanker. Available at: http://watchdog.org/130420/ ms-gulf-coast-lng-boom. Accessed July 19, 2017.

49. Smith Hopkins J. Plans for Sparrows Point terminal scrapped. *Baltimore Sun*. September 30, 2013. Available at: http://www.baltimoresun.com/business/bs-bz-sparrows-point-lng-terminal-scrapped-20130930-story.html. Accessed March 11, 2017.

50. Liquefied natural gas: bubbling up. *The Economist*. May 31, 2014. Available at: http://www. economist.com/news/business/21603030-international-gas-market-developing-buyers-will-gain-more-sellers-bubbling-up. Accessed March 11, 2017.

51. US Energy Information Administration. Effect of increased levels of liquefied natural gas exports on US energy markets. 2014. Available: https://www.eia.gov/analysis/requests/fe. Accessed March 11, 2017.

52. Stanton EA, Ackerman F, Comings T, Knight P, Vitolo T, Hausman E. *Will LNG Exports Benefit the United States Economy?* Cambridge, MA; Synapse Energy Economics; 2013.

53. Montgomery WD, Tuladhar S. Macroeconomic impacts of LNG exports from the United States. 2013. Available at: http://www.nera.com/publications/archive/2013/macroeconomic-impacts-of-lng-exports-from-the-united-states.html. Accessed September 4, 2016.

54. Baron R, Bernstein P, Montgomery W, Tuladhar S. *Updated Macroeconomic Impacts of LNG Exports From the United States*. Washington, DC: NERA Economic Consulting; 2014.

55. Ebinger C, Massy K, Avasarala G. *Liquid Markets: Assessing the Case for US Exports of Lique-fied Natural Gas. Policy Brief 12-01*. Washington, DC: The Brookings Institution; 2012.

56. Deloitte. Made in America: economic impact of LNG exports from the United States. 2016. Available at: http://www2.deloitte.com/us/en/pages/energy-and-resources/articles/made-in-america-the-economic-impact-of-lng-exports-from-the-united-states.html. Accessed September 4, 2016.

57. Treyz F, Brooks R, Nystrom S, Kig B, Cook C, Morton C. *The Macroeconomic Impact of LNG Exports: Integrating the GPCM® Natural Gas Model and the PI+® Regional Model*. Washington, DC: Regional Economic Models (REMI); 2015.

58. Palti-Guzman L. Gas under pressure: the United States is ready to export LNG, but does the world want it? *Foreign Affairs*. January 8, 2016. Available at: https://www.foreignaffairs.com/ articles/united-states/2016-01-08/gas-under-pressure. Accessed March 11, 2017.

10

IMPROVING THE HEALTH
AND SAFETY OF INDOOR
LIVING SPACES

Typical U.S. residents spend 90 percent or more of their time indoors. The youngest, oldest, disabled, and other especially vulnerable populations spend even more. It follows that indoor environments should be at least as healthy and safe as outdoor ones. Two building environments, in particular, are important to residents and their local governments: their homes and schools. A home remains the largest asset for most people; it should be protected and enhanced to increase its desirability. A good school system with superior instruction and attractive facilities is an asset to residents and the community as a whole. Indeed, we know from experience that realtors try to sell good houses in attractive neighborhoods near schools with excellent reputations.

The public expects planners and public health practitioners, as well as teachers, the police, firemen, sanitation workers, and everyone else in local government to support their quality of life and their assets. When residents do not get what they want, some become nasty. The following three exchanges, paraphrased and toned down from the actual ones, were between members of the public and planning, public health, and education officials and were witnessed by or told to the authors:

Homeowner to member of the planning board: I spent nearly three-quarters of a million dollars on our dream home in [town]. Your board members are crazy. How could you [members of the planning board] permit the farmer across the road to use liquid manure as a fertilizer? I can't escape the stink, unless I run the air conditioning all the time. Even then, the smell permeates everything. It is inexcusable! We have the right to enjoy our property. If I tried to sell it now, I would lose a lot of money.

Employee to local health officer: My office building is a [bleeping] health hazard. It is either too cold or too warm. We have no windows; the thermostats do not work. I have to keep extra jackets, a fan, and a space heater in the office. We are all catching colds and God knows what else from working here. You [health officer] need to intervene and order them to fix this.

Homeowner to local school board: You are talking about raising my property tax to pay for unproven so-called green investments in the school. What are you going to do when the green roof fails or when the solar panels don't pay for themselves? Your job is to hire good teachers to teach our children, not to use the school system to advocate your environmental ideology using our money.

This chapter focuses on three sets of tools for planners and health officials faced with challenging building environment issues:

- Building and zoning codes
- Indoor air quality tools
- Green building practices and sustainable development

Zoning codes date to antiquity, with mentions in the Code of Hammurabi, the Bible, and Roman texts. The second set of tools focuses on indoor air quality because we believe it to be a critical indoor public health risk. The green building tool set is of much more recent origin and attempts to subsume the first two.

The city of New Orleans, Louisiana, is featured in this chapter because of the human health and land use disaster that followed Hurricane Katrina in August 2005. Officials in federal, state, and especially local agencies, as well as private organizations, have made ongoing efforts to help rebuild the city using the tools described in this chapter and others. We review the overall effort for context but focus on two completed projects that are about 7 miles (a 15-minute car ride) apart in two of the most devastated areas of the city. One is a widely publicized housing development associated with actor Brad Pitt; the second is the rebuilding of an elementary school that had 2 feet of water in it after Katrina.

We deliberately resisted the temptation to feature some of the most famous green buildings constructed around the world in this chapter. Although these buildings are truly amazing and many people can visit them, no one lives in them and few people work in them.[1,2] Instead, this chapter is about places where people live and go to school, not places they dream about and may be fortunate to visit.

Building and Zoning Codes

Reading a building or zoning code is not fun. They may be long and difficult to understand, particularly in urban areas. But if you need to find out what you must do to make building on a site acceptable to a local government, then you need to read these codes and follow them closely. It is prudent to remember that local building and zoning codes are not suggestions; they are administrative law. Consider the example of building codes under the Code of Hammurabi (1754 BC), one based on the eye-for-an-eye principle. If someone was killed because his house fell on him, the code required that the builder be put to death. While perhaps an extreme mode of building code enforcement, it certainly sent an unequivocal message. Thus, we have a simple recommendation for those wishing to build: hire an expert and be sure they follow up-to-date local building codes.

Zoning ordinances control land use, and building codes focus on health and safety. The vast majority of cities, boroughs, and small towns have both. Houston, Texas, the major American city that does not have zoning, actually has a lot of regulations that look like and function like zoning.[3] Local governments have the authority to write the codes as they choose, although there are exceptions. For example, it is no longer permitted to write a zoning ordinance or code that directly or indirectly excludes certain populations (e.g., blacks, Jews).[4] See Chapter 2 for more on the use of zoning for this purpose.

A zoning ordinance is intended to prevent a land use that is incompatible with surrounding land uses. A residential area is not supposed to have a cement plant, junkyard, landfill, or metal fabricating plant located in the middle of it, although there are on-the-ground examples that belie that principle. The idea is that specialized land use zones allow each land use category to flourish. Thus, urban places typically separate residential districts from commercial zones. These designations address building use, size, height, and where different parts of the facility can be located, including parking and signs. Cities will have more types of zones, including many types of residential districts, from relatively low-density (single-family) ones to high-density multi-story apartment districts. Some cities have one or more mixed office–residential districts, with business zoning ranging from neighborhood stores to densely used downtown commercial centers. Cities with manufacturing bases will have a light-manufacturing zone where nuisance-related problems such as noise, odors, smoke, vibration, and visible emissions are prohibited. Other manufacturing zones will be set aside for production and waste management facilities.

The first example in this chapter quoted an irate resident who purchased his dream home adjacent to a farm that used liquid manure. It provides a clear illustration of how major clashes can occur when an agricultural district has been opened up to residential activities. In our example, farming had been the dominant land use and the courts decided that the farmers were entitled to use liquid manure. The newcomers lost their court challenge, but in the end the parties agreed upon how they could coexist.

A typical zoning case is not about the smell of manure; it is about parking—how much is required and where it is to be located (or not located) on the site. Stormwater management is another typical issue, often leading to setting aside land for stormwater capture.

Developers may seek variances from the zoning ordinance, arguing extenuating circumstances. For example, in the first author's neighborhood, a developer wanted to build two dozen condominiums on a site that held three large single-family homes. There was little opposition to the proposed development because some of the residents wanted to sell their large houses and move into the proposed smaller units. The zoning variance was not approved, however, until the developer agreed to move the parking from the front of the proposed units to the rear and add landscaping to improve the appearance of the new development.

Building codes are about human health and safety, and a key point is that they represent minimal requirements. Occupancy is a standard part of a building code, requiring that the developer indicate how many are going to live in the housing unit. Similar information is required from storeowners but translated into number and placement of entrances and exits. The code sets forth not only type of occupancy but also type of construction and materials used, maximum area per floor, numbers of exits, fire-resistant attributes, means of access and egress, and engineered systems. In some places, building codes are remarkably detailed, specifying foundations, roof types, stairs, energy efficiency, drainage, swimming pool requirements, requirements in anticipation of natural hazards (earthquakes, hurricanes, tsunamis), storage of flammable materials, methods of installation, and qualifications of the installers.[5] During a period when the first author was flying quite a bit, he wanted to know if there were building codes for tall structures along the takeoff and landing paths in two cities. There were codes.

Building codes are normally the focus of architects, engineers, builders, and their attorneys. As a project develops, however, many others (manufacturers, inspectors, landscapers, environmental analysts, insurance agents, and occupants) become parties to the implementation of requirements. Building codes normally are a combination of prescriptions that builders must follow and/or performance levels that can be met in a variety of ways.

Some have characterized zoning ordinances and building codes as rigid constraints on development and personal property. The reality is that they are essential to prevent inappropriate land use decisions and buildings that would not be even minimally protective of residents, workers, and visitors. Can these legal documents be made less rigid? Form-based codes (see Chapter 2) are intended to address this issue[6] but they require added design costs, planning, and other activities. In 2016, only about 3 percent of the 20,000 U.S. municipalities had form-based codes, the codes that best support the intentions of many green building practices.[7]

Indoor Air Quality

Although people primarily live indoors, the priority of the federal and state governments to date has been on outdoor air quality. Zoning ordinances, building codes, and green building practice all contribute to clean indoor air quality, yet the World Health Organization notes that indoor air pollution remains the "greatest environmental health risk"[8] and the literature lists more than 100 agents of concern in indoor air.[9] Here we focus on nine biological, chemical, and physical agents. They are listed in alphabetical order, not in order of public or worker risk.[10,11]

1. Allergens, molds, animal dander, and other biological agents, including *Legionella*, compose a large set of biological agents that are common in the indoor environment and cause health impacts ranging from red eyes to death.
2. Asbestos is a carcinogen, used in shingles, floor tiles, and as insulation around boilers and radiators, and it must be carefully removed during rebuilding.
3. Carbon dioxide is produced by human exhaling and is used as an indicator of poor ventilation in an indoor environment.
4. Carbon monoxide is a gas that produces breathing problems and at high concentrations causes death.
5. Lead is a widely used chemical found in older homes with lead paint and is a serious threat to young children with rapidly growing central nervous systems.
6. Nitrogen dioxide is a gas produced by poor quality gas stoves that can produce respiratory symptoms.
7. Radon is a gas caused by the decay of radium, is estimated by the U.S. Environmental Protection Agency (EPA) to be the major cause of death in the indoor environment in the United States, and its cancer-producing impacts are multiplied in tobacco smokers.
8. Tobacco smoke is a toxic byproduct that primarily impacts smokers but also is a threat to nonsmokers as secondhand smoke.
9. Volatile organic compounds include a wide variety of products found in paint and paint removers, lacquers, cleaning supplies and other solvents, copier ink, glue, pesticides, permanent markers, and many others that cause allergic reactions, drowsiness, illnesses, and poisoning.

The intent of this section is to highlight some of the tools that are available to cope with the multitude of indoor air threats. At the high end, some very sophisticated computer modeling has been conducted in regard to the spread of airborne agents. For example, the first author had a good friend who seemed to have more than the average of two to three colds a year. After having him keep a diary, we hypothesized that his part-time work as a bartender was responsible for undermining his immune system. We were able to measure the size and ventilation of the bar and estimate a distribution of the number of smokers in the bar (33 during his typical shift). He also lived with a chain smoker. Using an air-dispersion model, we estimated that he was inhaling the equivalent of more than two dozen cigarettes a day and was violating the national outdoor ambient air quality standard for particulates by a factor of 10. Within six months, he quit this job, moved into his own apartment, and felt better. The cause-and-effect relationship between his indoor air environment and his health may be debatable, but the model certainly helped us both understand more about secondhand tobacco smoke. The same kind of estimates

Table 10.1. Selected Items for Teachers from U.S. Environmental Protection Agency Checklist Regarding Indoor Air Quality

Category With Possible Answers of Yes, No, or Not Applicable

1. General cleanliness
    1a. Ensured rooms are dusted and vacuumed regularly.
    1b. Ensured rooms are free of clutter.
    1c. Ensured that trash is removed daily.
    1d. Ensured that no food is stored in classroom overnight.
    1e. Ensured that animal food is stored in tightly sealed containers.
    1f. Ensured room is free of pests and vermin.
    1g. Used unscented, school-approved cleaners and air fresheners in rooms.
2. Animals in the classroom (7 items)
3. Drain trap in the classroom (3 items)
4. Excess moisture in classrooms (7 items)
5. Thermal comfort
    5a. Ensured moderate temperature (should generally be 72°F to 76°F).
    5b. Ensured there are no signs of draftiness.
    5c. Ensured that students are not seated in direct sunlight.
    5d. Ensured that indoor humidity is maintained at acceptable levels (between 30 percent and 60 percent).
6. Ventilation (7 items)
7. Educational supplies (art, science industrial/vocational; 11 items)
8. Local exhaust fans (4 items)
9. Locker room (5 items)

Source: Based on U.S. Environmental Protection Agency.[13]

have been done for viruses, lead, asbestos, and other places where humans congregate—for example, in aircraft.[12]

As simulation tools require a great deal of specialized knowledge, we focus instead on a simpler set of tools that provide valuable insights about and solutions to indoor air exposures. Checklists have been prepared for buildings in general and for schools in particular. The checklist tool for schools includes separate questions for teachers, administrative staff, health officers and school nurses, and school officials. Each of checklists has a different focus and is supported by fact sheets and references. The one for health officers has a focus on maintaining student health records and health education. There is also one that focuses on the roof, ground level, bathrooms, combustion appliances, and other engineered parts of the grounds. All of these checklists are useful.

The first author prefers the checklist for teachers. Table 10.1 shows the major subheadings (reduced from 56 items) and the sections on general cleanliness and thermal comfort. Table 10.2 is a similar reduction of the checklist for health officers and school nurses.

These straightforward questions can be used to determine if there is a serious problem or looming problem that needs to be addressed, sometimes with follow-up analysis with

Table 10.2. Selected Items From U.S. Environmental Protection Agency Checklist for Health Officers and School Nurses

Category Followed by Answers of Yes, No, or Not Applicable

1. Maintaining student health
   1a. Completed health records for each student.
   1b. Updated health records, as appropriate.
   1c. Obtained necessary information about student allergies and other health factors.
   1d. Developed a system to log health complaints.
   1e. Monitored trends in health complaints.
   1f. Investigated potential causes of health complaints.
   1g. Ensured that the school prohibits smoking.
   1h. Noted any new warm-blooded animals introduced into classrooms.
   1i. Reviewed and understood indicators of IAQ-related problems.
2. Health, IAQ, and hygiene education
   2a. Educated students and staff about the importance of good hygiene.
   2b. Arranged individual instruction/counseling where necessary.
   2c. Developed information and education programs for parents and staff.
   2d. Established an information and counseling program for smokers.
   2e. Provided literature on smoking and secondhand smoke.
   2f. Educated school staff, students, and parents on the link between IAQ and health.
3. Health officer's office
   3a. Ensured the ventilation system operates properly and supplies adequate quantities of outdoor air.
   3b. Ensured that air filters are clean and properly installed.
   3c. Ensured that air supply pathways are clear of any obstructions.
   3d. Determined that health office air is separated from the ventilation system to avoid affecting other areas of the school.

Source: Based on U.S. Environmental Protection Agency.[14]
Note: IAQ=indoor air quality.

air dispersion models such as the one described earlier. If an unacceptable exposure is documented, the following options are available to reduce the risk:

- Remove existing agents, such as asbestos, lead paint, and volatile organic substances.
- Warn occupants to monitor stoves, heating equipment, and other appliances that can emit toxic substances and catch on fire.
- Filter the air to capture noxious contaminants.
- Ventilate to dilute concentrations of noxious air contaminants, especially when new rugs, upholstery, and other furniture and equipment are added.
- Remove and/or routinely clean areas where contaminants are found, such as rugs, furniture, windowsills, and any other horizontal surfaces.
- Monitor for nonvisible agents, such as radon, and remediate unacceptable exposures with reliable engineered solutions.
- Add vegetation that can absorb carbon dioxide and yet will not cause allergic reactions, while removing plants that may cause allergic reactions.

- Educate occupants about the risks and management strategies for maintaining a healthy indoor environment.

Green Building Practices and Sustainable Development

The EPA reports[15] that buildings account for impacts associated with the following:

- 39 percent of U.S. energy use
- 39 percent of U.S. carbon dioxide emissions
- 68 percent of total electricity consumption
- 12 percent of U.S. fresh water use
- Indoor environmental exposures where people spend the vast majority of their time

To reduce the impact of buildings, the EPA has embraced green building, defined as "maximizing the efficiency with which buildings and their sites use resources—energy, water, and materials—while minimizing building impacts on human health and the environment, throughout the complete building life cycle—from siting, design, and construction to operation, renovation, and reuse."[15]

Green building practices existed long before the green building label appeared in the 21st century. For example, the Flatiron Building[16] in New York City is located between 22nd and 23rd streets in Manhattan (about 1.1 miles south of the Empire State Building). It is famous for its triangular shape, but when it opened in 1902, its deep-set windows were designed to shade the interior from the sun. Rockefeller Center, a world-famous 1932 Art Deco building on Fifth Avenue between 49th and 50th streets (about 1.4 miles north of the Empire State Building) installed sky gardens and operable windows.[17] During the 1970s, in the wake of the oil embargo, architects, planners, and health-conscious individuals began devising energy-saving building strategies. These strategies were enhanced during the 1990s to ultimately become today's green building practices. Successful programs are those that connect efforts to protect the outdoor environment as well as the indoor one. In alphabetical order, these programs focus on the following:

- Increasing energy efficiency
- Increasing sustainable development
- Increasing water use efficiency
- Minimizing toxic substance use and exposure
- Reducing indoor air pollution
- Reducing waste
- Using building materials that are less environmentally destructive

In essence, a green building is a structure that is resource-efficient and protective of human health and safety throughout its lifecycle, and its envelope extends to the surrounding area, which may be as small as the grounds surrounding the facility but often means the surrounding neighborhood.[18,19] Green building practices are directly related to sustainable development in that their objective is to continue to support a healthy economy while at the same time providing a high quality of life for humans and protecting natural ecosystems in perpetuity.

Green building rating systems include the U.S. Green Building Council's Leadership in Energy and Environmental Design (LEED)[20] and the Green Building Initiative's Green Globes.[21] Space does not permit us to explore the details of these rating systems, but a considerable amount has been published about them.[22,23] All of us can visit showcase green buildings, but we can also incorporate green building practices into our own homes by building smaller, incorporating solar panels, using more efficient appliances, installing energy-efficient windows, and more. We encourage readers to look into life-cycle assessment of the green building process, from original design or purchase, through operation, and finally closing and disposal.

The EPA has created toolkits for the components of green building and sustainable development.[24,25] Each of the toolkits begins with an introduction to the subject matter, then provides an assessment tool followed by description of how communities can build an action plan for green building and implement it. The toolkits include the following:

- Energy Conservation and Atmospheric Quality
- General Green Building Resources
- Indoor Environmental Air Quality
- Material and Resource Conservation
- Sustainable Sites and Responsible Land Use Development
- Water Efficiency, Conservation, and Management

Table 10.3 summarizes codes and other regulations and offers recommendations to improve air quality in neighborhoods with green building and sustainable design practices.

Case Studies: Green Building in New Orleans Post-Katrina

Chapters 5 through 9 focused on 15 tools applied to formidable issues across the United States. It would be difficult, however, to find a major city that has been challenged more by adversity during the 21st century than New Orleans. This chapter focuses on the residential and school indoor environments in that city, but it also shows how building and implementing plans requires walking a tight rope between making stakeholders happy and making good decisions.

Table 10.3. Sample Air Quality Checklist Questions From the U.S. Environmental Protection Agency Sustainable Design and Green Building Toolkit

Questions About Local Ordinances and Codes	Potential Environmental Management Tools
Neighborhood Air Quality	
Are there requirements for dust management on the construction site to prevent offsite migration of dust?	• Dust management specifications
Does the construction equipment need to use clean diesel fuel or alternative fuels to reduce greenhouse emissions?	• Clean diesel initiatives • Clean construction initiatives
Heat Island	
Are there requirements to minimize heat generated from rooftops? Parking areas? Streets and driveways?	• Green roof specifications • Green parking specifications • Green street specifications • Low reflectance roof coverings • Permeable pavement specifications
Are there incentives for maintaining or restoring tree canopies?	• Tree requirements (native species, maintenance requirements) • Canopy requirements
Indoor Air Quality	
Are there minimum requirements that protect indoor air quality and minimize energy loss?	• Codes have most recent American National Standards Institute standards for residential (62.2) and commercial (62.1) structures
Are there requirements for controlling indoor particulates?	• Requirements for particulate control in the indoor environment, tracking at the entry level, and construction specifications for inside homes
Are smoking bans in place?	• Smoking bans • Minimum building setbacks for smoking areas from the building entrance
Does indoor air delivery promote occupant health?	• Monitoring devices on outdoor delivery systems • Ozone-removing filters • Prevention of air emissions from the garage flowing into the house • Radon control, where needed • Construction specifications for homes • Vapor barriers as needed

Source: Adapted from U.S. Environmental Protection Agency.[24]

When Katrina hit the New Orleans area on August 29, 2005, hundreds of thousands of residents were displaced, property damage was estimated at over $100 billion, and residents had to live with the reality that parts of the region would be unoccupied for the foreseeable future. About 150,000 homes, schools, and other buildings were destroyed or severely damaged. Approximately four-fifths of the population of approximately 500,000 residents left before the storm. Nearly 100,000 were left in the city because they had no method of egress and thereby faced a 10- to 20-foot-high storm surge.[26,27]

New Orleans's vulnerability was not a surprise. The city had been losing its natural environmental buffers for decades, first slowly and then at an increased rate. The city was clearly vulnerable to a major storm and had borne the brunt of several. New Orleans also had a large vulnerable population living below the poverty line before the hurricane, and they were disproportionately located in the neighborhoods most vulnerable to the storm surge and structural failures. As expected, the American Red Cross, the Salvation Army, and other religious and not-for-profit groups entered to provide food, shelter, and immediate assistance when the storm abated.

Shortly after the hurricane, Mayor Ray Nagin established a "Bring New Orleans Back" Commission to develop and implement plans for rebuilding and repopulating the city.[28] The Commission's vision for the city illustrates how stakeholders injected human health and safety, economic and environmental health, and social conditions into the planning process. The Commission focused its suggestions on four plans:

1. Flood and stormwater protection to include perimeter and internal levies, pumping and gates to control water, and coastal wetland restoration
2. Transportation improvements, such as high-speed light rail with connections to the airport, to Baton Rouge (the state capital), and to the Gulf Coast, and greater emphasis placed on walking and bicycles
3. Parks and open space that would serve the needs of residents and serve as internal stormwater management control
4. Neighborhood rebuilding focused around neighborhood centers

The Commission generated multiple reports focusing on culture, economic development, education, government effectiveness, health and social services, infrastructure, levees and flood protection, criminal justice, public transit, and urban planning. Their efforts reflected an immediate response to the crisis.

In contrast to the Commission's work, Costanza and colleagues[29] presented an intermediate- to long-term vision of rebuilding New Orleans consistent with what planners and public health officials typically do. They called for local officials to recognize the reality that much of this city is at or below sea level and sinking further. It follows, they argue, that it is not logical nor is it sustainable to rebuild back to the same pattern that previously existed. The authors suggest that the current land uses in these areas be replaced with wetlands, and/or structures that are adapted to flooding by raising them or floating them and placing only noncritical elements on lower levels of structures. They suggest using the attributes of the Mississippi River system to rebuild the coast rather than trying to direct the flow of the river, which has only increased the city's vulnerability. This and other papers and studies also called for rebuilding the social capital of the city by investing in diversity, tolerance, fairness, and justice. The Rockefeller Foundation and others committed to helping with rebuilding New Orleans along these tenets.[30,31]

In November 2005, the U.S. Green Building Council embraced the challenge of the post-Katrina disaster with a charrette at its annual conference in Atlanta, Georgia.[32] The meeting included 160 participants, approximately 20 percent from the New Orleans area, who had backgrounds in planning, water resources, engineering, and architecture. The principles they articulated point directly at rebuilding around environmental, economic, and equity-based redevelopment solutions. The 10 principles are presented in the same order as in the report of the charrette (Table 10.4).

This charrette concluded, as have others, that although it is possible to rebuild New Orleans back to its former land-use pattern, it would neither be desirable nor sustainable in the face of continuing threats from environmental hazard. Rather than trying to conquer nature, the authors suggest that green building practices increase the probability of withstanding another storm and recovering from it, as well as recognizing the diversity and multipurpose living environments that have historically characterized New Orleans.

Much has been written about the precursors of the Katrina disaster and post-Katrina responses. Olshansky and Johnson's book,[33] published in 2010, captures the essential land use and human health planning challenges. After describing the $100 billion to $150 billion in damages, the authors reviewed the Bring New Orleans Back Commission and later efforts to organize the city's redevelopment. They characterize the Commission as hindered by a lack of data and an inability to access stakeholders. They then describe redevelopment efforts by the federal government, the Urban Land Institute, and the American Planning Association, as well as the State of Louisiana.

Table 10.4. U.S. Green Building Council Principles for Rebuilding New Orleans

1. Respect the rights of all citizens of New Orleans (allow displaced residents to return to neighborhoods of their choice).
2. Restore natural protection of the greater New Orleans region (manage and restore the ecosystem to protect the area.
3. Implement an inclusive planning process (build the process with local stakeholders).
4. Value diversity in New Orleans (encourage diversity of land use, ethnicity/race, socioeconomic status).
5. Protect the City of New Orleans (build a protective infrastructure using both natural and engineering approaches).
6. Embrace smart development (rebuild compact neighborhoods around schools and provide multiple transit options).
7. Honor the past; build for the future (honor the city's unique history, but build modern, safe, and healthy buildings).
8. Provide for passive survivability (build facilities and neighborhoods so that people can survive in the event of a crisis or breakdown).
9. Foster locally owned, sustainable businesses (support local business in regard to building sustainable contributions).
10. Focus on the long term (emphasize long-term objectives).

Source: Based on U.S. Green Building Council (2005).[32(p4)]

Olshansky and Johnson carefully examined the Unified New Orleans Plan,[31] noting that it was approved by more than 90 percent of the participants in the planning process. The authors assert that the plan was widely supported because all of the priorities represented by the participants were incorporated into the final report. The authors are skeptical of the outcome, however, contending that is highly unlikely that many of the approved outcomes will be implemented because of their cost. They pose an interesting question: is it better to gain a consensus and have an approved plan, or is it better to have a realistic set of projects to work on? This tension is present in many land-use and public health plans, and is simply more apparent in this particular case.

To set the context for the two indoor case studies in this chapter, we briefly summarize what happened after the Katrina event. By September 5, 2005, about a week after Katrina struck, downtown New Orleans began to once again receive electrical power. One day after that, the critical Port of New Orleans was opened. The U.S. Army Corps of Engineers began rebuilding dozens of levees and, by early October 2005, water and sewage service was operational.

Despite the speed with which infrastructure returned to the city, the political, economic, and social rebuilding processes have been much slower to return. Various discussions occurred in the U.S. Congress about the federal government's responsibility to the New Orleans area. It was in the city's favor that this area has some unique social and cultural attributes and a history of re-electing its congressional representatives for many years. In other words, the region's representatives sit in some powerful congressional committee positions.

New Orleans has a long history of racial and income segregation. How much effort should be made to break this pattern as part of the rebuilding process? If this was an explicit goal, how would it be done and how would it be paid for? Heated debates arose for and against rebuilding patterns—whether to place hotels and housing for the affluent in the most flood-prone areas or to use resources to rebuild housing for individuals of more modest means. It is not irrational to argue that the former option would be better for New Orleans in the long run as hotels, restaurants, and recreation facilities would have more money to build at or above code for flood prevention. These facilities would create jobs and income that presumably would trickle down to the poorer segments of the population. On the other hand, such a policy meant driving out historically poor populations that had lived in the flood-prone areas for many decades, and it sent not-too-subtle messages that money interests were more important than equity ones.

The Indoor Residential Environment

There was massive damage to residential structures in New Orleans and environs when levees failed allowing billions of gallons of water into the area. Temporary housing was built and work-arounds allowed parts of the city to return to a new normal. Eleven years after the hurricane, the new normal is still evolving. The population was 485,000 according the U.S. Census of 2000, and after Katrina it fell more than 50 percent to 230,000. By July 2015, the city's population was estimated at 387,000, or about 80 percent of the pre-event population.

A great deal of housing was rebuilt and new residences have been added to the city's housing stock. The least-damaged areas were the initial focus of rebuilding and then gradually attention was shifted to the areas near the levees. Tons of debris and abandoned cars had to be removed before any new building could be done. Some people stayed in the upper floors of multi-unit facilities. The ground floors were stripped, reinforced, and rebuilt. Roof damage was extensive, and the authors' colleagues who live and teach in New Orleans described these as "blue roof" neighborhoods because blue tarpaulins were set on top of damaged roofs to hold out the rain. Some had a supply of buckets and other equipment to capture rainwater. These makeshift solutions were challenged by the typical wet weather in the New Orleans area.

The Federal Emergency Management Agency (FEMA) brought in temporary housing after the storm, but some of these units subjected the population to unacceptably high levels of indoor contaminants. Others leaked and were so unsuitable that they were abandoned. Overall, the devastation in a good part of New Orleans was unprecedented in scale, albeit not in deaths (see Galveston in Chapter 6), and the basics of providing shelter, water, and energy; protecting human health; and economic recovery all had to be addressed without delay.

Multiple housing projects were started in New Orleans, yet a disproportionate amount of attention has been focused around relatively few units in the heavily damaged lower Ninth Ward area, which sits adjacent to the Mississippi River. Actor Brad Pitt founded the "Make It Right" Foundation, an effort to build 150 units of modest housing in a greener style. Part of the process was a competition that sought out the most environmentally friendly designs. The six finalists were chosen from 125 entries: New Orleans (2), New York City (3), and Chicago. The videos finalists submitted addressed affordability, health, and energy use, including trees and trellises to cool buildings, a priority in the heat and humidity of New Orleans.[34]

As of early 2016, more than 100 houses had been completed at the site, about 5 miles east of the Superdome and 4.2 miles from the French Quarter. Homeowners could select from 21 designs, including duplexes and single-family homes. They choose combinations of paints, cabinets, countertops, and flooring, with an average unit size of about 1,400 square feet. The developers adopted the LEED Platinum certification standards, the highest level for this kind of building, and the Global Green project offered audits to the homes. The new homes included solar panels and countertops made of recycled materials with the goal of having energy bills only one-third of conventional homes of the same size. They used building materials that release no or few distressing agents with an explicit goal of improving indoor air quality to reduce asthma symptoms. For human health and safety, the homes were elevated 5 to 8 feet above the ground, with exits to the roof so people would not be trapped in a future flood event, which many unfortunately were in the aftermath of Katrina.[35]

Not surprisingly, not everyone praised the green building housing efforts in New Orleans. In the case of the Brad Pitt–sponsored project, Doggett[36] praised the idea of green building in general but pointed to issues with the structural insulated panels. These are vulnerable to high water infiltration and will not be durable in the moist New Orleans environment. Alexander[37] reported that some of the wood used in the Make It Right Homes was rotting and needed to be replaced. The builders responded that they were investigating and would replace any defects. These reports underscore the fact that we have insufficient studies to evaluate the long-term performance of all residential green building practices. We also do not have sufficient data from a broad spectrum of people to know what homeowners living in modest homes think about their green enviroments.[38] For New Orleans, the green building of residential housing is a positive attribute to attract new interest in the city.[39,40] We cannot predict, however, whether the results of these efforts will improve the quality of life for the new homeowners over the coming decades.

The Indoor Educational Environment

In July 2006, The Education Committee of the Bring New Orleans Back Commission documented the status of New Orleans public education system before and immediately after Hurricane Katrina as follows:

> Prior to Katrina, Orleans Parish ranked among the lowest performing of large urban school districts nation-wide and was facing significant financial problems.[41(p2)]

Indeed, before the storm, Orleans Parish had an outstanding debt of $370 million and its finances were taken over by a private contractor. After the storm, the contractor estimated that Orleans Parish needed an additional $1 billion to rebuild the school system's deteriorated structures. In addition, of the district's 117 schools, 68 were classified as unacceptable for student performance and 44 were performing below the state average. With more than 90 percent of the schools in trouble, an independent body, the Recovery School District, took over their management with the primary goal of raising the quality of student performance. The Education Committee of the Bring New Orleans Back Commission set forth ambitious goals for New Orleans schools, including, "achieving top 10 percent performance in the United States across key measures," which required "creat[ing] schools and learning-centered environments that meet the academic, emotional, and social needs of all students."[41(p2)]

Hurricanes Katrina (August) and Rita (September) damaged 28 to 40 of these 117 schools beyond repair. Since about 80 percent of the resident population left the area, the school system did not have to immediately rebuild all the schools. Students went to existing undamaged schools and to makeshift facilities. In January 2006, 9,000 students were enrolled in the New Orleans school system, in what were now mostly charter schools operated by their own boards and with the authority to hire their principal, staff, and teachers. The charter schools were funded by the taxpayers and required to meet performance criteria to retain their charter and their funding.

The 33-page Education Committee report had little to say about the indoor physical environment of the schools. For example, it states that

> well equipped, well-maintained facilities: all stakeholders would like to see new learner-centered buildings to replace those that have been damaged. In all the discussions, stakeholders [recognized] a need for better maintenance of school property.[41(p10–11)]

Indeed, nearly the entire report focused on the school system's objectives, control of the system, and accountability. Relatively little was said about the physical plant, most likely because the committee's mandate was organizing the school system. Our point is that a large amount of money was going to be spent on the physical plant leaving professionals in design, planning, and healthy school environments to fill the void. *Time Magazine* said, "No organization is doing more to green New Orleans."[40]

In 2015, Jewson[42] reported that New Orleans had completed 19 new schools as part of a $1.8-billion school rebuilding plan funded by FEMA. Many other schools were almost complete; others were being renovated, 29 were being refurbished, some were demolished, and some remain boarded up awaiting decisions. By academic year 2013–2014, New Orleans public school enrollment was 46,000 students, lower than the 65,000 pre-Katrina number but much higher than the 9,000 reported by the Education Committee in 2006.

City residents supported the plan for addressing the public school issues with a $150-million tax. Dobard[43] led the Renew School District Board beginning in 2012 and noted that nearly all the physical projects would be completed by 2018. Collectively, students were performing better than before the storm. Their state test scores were up and the high-school graduation rate rose from 54 percent in 2004 to 73 percent in 2014. Superintendent Dobard[43] characterized the traditional school district as a "cruise ship" compared with the Recovery School Districts that were "speedboats"—nimble, allowing the school districts to quickly shift to meet needs and take advantage of opportunities. Chieppo[44] praised New Orleans for improving state test scores and graduation rates, but he questioned whether there was too much emphasis on college preparation and not enough on vocational education. The *Green Money Journal* also addressed this topic.[45]

The Andrew H. Wilson School

The Andrew H. Wilson School was chosen as a model high-performance school by the Recovery School District. Located about 2 miles southwest of the Superdome and

3.7 miles from the French Quarter, the original school dated from 1912 and an accessory building was added during the 1940s. In 2005, 2 feet of water seeped into the first floor, damaged the roof, and made the accessory building unusable. Rebuilding of this school sits within the context of the rebuilding of the entire city public school system,[46] part of a $1.8-billion reconstruction program. It is also presented here in the context of the third bullet point that opened this chapter: "You are talking about raising my property tax to pay for unproven so-called 'green' investments in the school."

The first author visited the Andrew H. Wilson School, located on General Pershing Street in the Broadmoor neighborhood of New Orleans. The school was intended to serve 540 students from pre-kindergarten to the eighth grade. It has 26 classrooms, a cafeteria, gym, art studio, computer lab, music and art rooms, library, and administrative offices. Although most schools have these attributes, the internal design is markedly different from other new schools that we have seen. It includes the following:

- Enhanced natural lighting provided by specially designed windows and a building envelope oriented to capture and use sunlight
- Enhanced acoustics in classrooms meant to focus sound within the room and exclude sound outside it
- Enhanced lighting with options for dimming and controlling glare, and color schemes that complement daylight
- Use of green construction materials, some of which are incorporated into the curriculum

As you approach the building or look at it on Google maps, you cannot miss the existing steep roof with terracotta red tile. An adjacent new building has a steep roof made of metal panels, and another has a low slope made of white modified bitumen. The net goal of the external design is to minimize any heat island effect, which is a major issue in New Orleans during the summer. Energy use is reduced by including photovoltaics on one roof, R-30 roof insulation and SRI-330 roof membranes on another, R-30 wall insulation, the use of low-e Argon windows that are clear to improve natural daylight, and other green outside features. The outside visible features are impressive and the indoor ones are no less so (Table 10.5).

The school was designed to meet LEED certification for schools in 2007 and we cannot possibly do justice to its positive interior green attributes. Outside, we examined the school's accessibility with regard to distance from public transportation (about 1.4 miles away), as well as access for the school bus system, auto parking, bicycle storage, the public library, nearest firehouse, and other services. This was important, as a laudable goal of the rebuild was to share the school's facilities with both the neighborhood and a YMCA (the latter was dropped because of a lack of space and cost).

The first author went to a public school, PS 53 in the South Bronx, which, like Andrew H. Wilson School, was originally built in 1912. PS 53 is a five-story brick and

Table 10.5. Selected Indoor Attributes of the Andrew H. Wilson School

1. Indoor environmental quality
   - Low use of volatile organic compound off-gassing paint, adhesives, and sealants
   - Classrooms acoustically insulated from other classrooms
2. Water resources
   - Rain gardens across the site
   - Permeable pavers
   - Rainwater collection tank
   - Underground water percolation technology and retention areas
3. Material reuse
   - Reuse of 90 percent of the existing building
   - Recycled rubber gym flooring and plastic benches
   - Use of recycled concrete
   - 80 percent of construction waste recycled
   - Six oak trees on the site restored
4. Energy use
   - Reflective roofing that reduces solar heat gain
   - Solar-driven hot water system in the kitchen
   - Efficient Deming lamps that respond to occupant density
   - Building designed to capture daylight

Source: Based on HMS Architects (2007).[47]

limestone structure. One of its teachers told the first author when he visited for the 100th year anniversary that "the school has tried to educate generations of mischievous boys like you in what has been a poor- or lower-middle-class area." Although PS 53 has been rehabilitated, now sporting more technology than it had during the early 1950s, it remains a typical, fairly sterile public school environment. Despite being located in a poor area of New Orleans, the Andrew H. Wilson School seems a forward-looking and exciting environment in which to learn, a school that increases the value of the neighborhood. Yet this amazing building has not led to better student performance (the school's overall student performance grade had fallen from D in 2012–2013 to F in 2013–2014). In February 2015, the existing charter for this school was cancelled and a new group took over. Although some local residents were upset, others were not.[48,49]

Final Thoughts

This book only dedicated one chapter to the indoor environment, but it is a critical topic because we spend so much of our time indoors. In fact, the most vulnerable among us spend nearly all their time indoors. Historically, building codes and zoning ordinances have been the legal mechanisms for setting standards about where different land uses are permitted and how the public is protected. Without them, we will face significant health and safety challenges in our living environments. No environmental health and safety challenge is more vital than air quality, which includes exposure to toxins, moisture, heat, and an array of exposures that can overwhelm people, especially those with pre-existing conditions. Green building programs promote sustainable development by making them more efficient, durable, and resilient, and more environmentally responsible. They create indoor environments that are healthy for residents, workers, students, and travelers.

References

1. The world's 10 coolest examples of "green buildings." Tomorrow's World. 2016. Available at: http://www.twnews.uk/the-worlds-10-coolest-examples-of-green-buildings. Accessed August 8, 2017.

2. Ten great examples of green building worldwide. Allianz. 2009. Available at: https://www.allianz.com/en/about_us/open-knowledge/topics/environment/articles/090717-ten-great-examples-of-green-building-worldwide.html. Accessed October 22, 2016.

3. Holeywell R. Forget what you've heard, Houston really does have zoning (sort of). The Urban Edge. 2015. Available at: https://urbanedge.blogs.rice.edu/2015/09/08/forget-what-youve-heard-houston-really-does-have-zoning-sort-of/#.WAubIi0rKUk. Accessed October 22, 2016.

4. Meck S. Zoning and anti-Semitism in the 1920s: the case of Cleveland Jewish Orphan Home v. Village of University Heights and its aftermath. *J Plan Hist*. 2005;4(2):91–128.

5. International Code Council. International Code Adoptions. 2016. Available at: http://www.iccsafe.org/about-icc/overview/international-code-adoptions. Accessed October 22, 2016.

6. Mammoser A. A crack in the code? Form-based codes. *Planning*. 2016;82(9):26–31.

7. *Form-Based Codes: A Step-by-Step Guide for Communities Acknowledgements Introduction: What Are Form-Based Codes?* Chicago, IL: Chicago Metropolitan Agency for Planning; 2012.

8. Brink S. WHO Report: Indoor air pollution is greatest environmental health risk. *National Geographic News*. March 27, 2014. Available at: http://news.nationalgeographic.com/news/2014/03/140325-world-health-organization-indoor-fuel-pollution-death. Accessed October 22, 2016.

9. *Report to the Congress: Indoor Air Pollution: An Emerging Health Problem*. Washington, DC: US Comptroller General; 1980.

10. Bas E. *Indoor Air Quality. A Guide for Facility Managers*. 2nd ed. New York, NY: Marcel Dekker Inc; 2004.

11. Spengler J, Samet J, McCarthy J. *Indoor Air Quality Handbook*. New York, NY: McGraw Hill; 2001.

12. Jones RM, Masago Y, Bartrand T, Haas CN, Nicas M, Rose JB. Characterizing the risk of infection from *Mycobacterium tuberculosis* in commercial passenger aircraft using quantitative microbial risk assessment. *Risk Anal*. 2009;29(3):355–365.

13. US Environmental Protection Agency. Teacher's classroom checklist from indoor air quality tools for schools. 2016. Available at: https://www.epa.gov/iaq-schools/teachers-classroom-checklist-indoor-air-quality-tools-schools. Accessed October 22, 2016.

14. US Environmental Protection Agency. Health officer and school nurse checklist from indoor air quality tools for schools. 2016. Available at: https://www.epa.gov/iaq-schools/health-officer-and-school-nurse-checklist-indoor-air-quality-tools-schools. Accessed October 22, 2016.

15. *EPA's Green Building Strategy EPA-100-F-08-073*. Washington, DC: US Environmental Protection Agency; 2008.

16. Gissen D. *Big and Green: Toward Sustainable Architecture in the 21st Century*. Princeton, NJ: Princeton Architectural Press; 2003.

17. Duempelmann S. *Flights of Imagination: Aviation, Landscape, Design*. Charlottesville, VA: University of Virginia Press; 2014.

18. Klöpffer W, Grahl B. *Life Cycle Assessment (LCA): A Guide to Best Practice*. Hoboken, NJ: Wiley; 2014.

19. US Environmental Protection Agency. Life cycle assessment: principles and practice. EPA/600/R-06/060, 200. 2006. Available at: https://cfpub.epa.gov/si/si_public_record_report.cfm?dirEntryId=155087. Accessed October 22, 2016.

20. US Green Building Council. Better buildings are our legacy. 2016. Available at: http://www.usgbc.org/leed. Accessed October 22, 2016.

21. Green Building Initiative. Green Globes Certification. 2014. Available at: https://www.thegbi.org/green-globes-certification. Accessed October 22, 2016.

22. Williams DE. *Sustainable Design: Ecology, Architecture, and Planning*. Hoboken, NJ: Wiley; 2007.

23. National Institute of Building Sciences. The Whole Building Design Guide. 2016. Available at: https://www.wbdg.org. Accessed October 22, 2016.

24. US Environmental Protection Agency. Best directory: building energy software tools. Psychrometric Analysis Design Suite. 2016. Available at: http://www.buildingenergysoftwaretools.com/software/psychrometric-analysis-design-suite. Accessed October 22, 2016.

25. *Sustainable Design and Green Building Toolkit: for Local Governments (EPA 904B10001)*. Washington, DC: US Environmental Protection Agency; 2013.

26. Brinkley D. *The Great Deluge: Hurricane Katrina, New Orleans, and the Mississippi Gulf Coast*. New York, NY: Harper Perennial; 2006.

27. Neufeld J. *A.D: New Orleans After the Deluge (Pantheon Graphic Novels)*. New York, NY: Pantheon; 2010.

28. Bring New Orleans Back Commission reports. 2006. Available at: http://www.columbia.edu/itc/journalism/cases/katrina/city_of_new_orleans_bnobc.html. Accessed October 22, 2016.

29. Costanza R, Mitsch WJ, Dya JW. A new vision for New Orleans and the Mississippi Delta: applying ecological economics and ecological engineering. *Front Ecol Environ*. 2006;4(9): 465–472.

30. The Rockefeller Foundation. New Orleans and the birth of urban resilience. 2016. Available at: https://www.rockefellerfoundation.org/new-orleans-birth-urban-resilience. Accessed October 22, 2016.

31. *The Unified New Orleans Plan: Citywide Strategic Recovery and Rebuilding Plan*. New Orleans, LA: City of New Orleans; 2007.

32. *The New Orleans Principles: Celebrating the Rich History of New Orleans Through Commitment to a Sustainable Future*. New Orleans, LA: US Green Building Council; 2005.

33. Olshansky R, Johnson L. *Clear as Mud: Planning for the Rebuilding of New Orleans*: Chicago, IL; Washington, DC: American Planning Association Press; 2010.

34. Rebuilding a better, greener New Orleans. *Today*. 2006. Available at: http://www.today.com/id/13892600/ns.today/t/rebui8lding-beter-greene#.WAuvZC0rKUk. Accessed October 22, 2016.

35. Global Green. Holy Cross Project in New Orleans. 2016. Available at: http://www.globalgreen.org/holy-cross-project-in-new-orleans. Accessed October 22, 2016.

36. Doggett MS. Making it green does not make it right. The Building Enclosure. 2014. Available at: https://builtenv.wordpress.com/2014/02/10/making-it-green-does-not-make-it-right. Accessed October 22, 2016.

37. Alexander H. Katrina victims say Brad Pitt's charity homes are already rotting. Chron. 2014. Available at: http://www.chron.com/news/houston-texas/texas/article/Katrina-victims-say-Brad-Pitt-s-charity-homes-are-5108452.php. Accessed October 22, 2016.

38. Abbaszadeh S, Zagreus L, Lehrer D, Huizenga C. Occupant satisfaction with indoor environmental quality in green buildings. *Cent Built Environ*. 2006;3(Lisbon):365–370.

39. Rebuilding Together New Orleans. Green rebuilding. 2016. Available at: http://www.rtno.org/get-educated/green. Accessed October 22, 2016.

40. Worland J. The green rebuilding of post-Katrina New Orleans. *TIME*. August 28, 2015. Available at: http://time.com/4014281/katrina-green-building. Accessed October 22, 2016.

41. *Rebuilding and Transforming: A Plan for Improving Public Education in New Orleans*. New Orleand, LA: Bring New Orleans Back Commission, Education Committee; 2006.

42. Jewson M. New Orleans has 19 new public schools as $1.8 billion building plan continues. *The Lens*. August 25, 2015. Available at: http://thelensnola.org/2015/08/25/new-orleans-has-19-new-public-schools-as-1-8-billion-building-plan-continues. Accessed October 22, 2016.

43. Dobard P. How we rebuilt New Orleans' schools "from scratch." *Education Week*. August 25, 2015. Available at: http://www.edweek.org/ew/articles/2015/08/26/how-we-rebuilt-new-orleans-schools-from.html. Accessed October 22, 2016.

44. Chieppo C. How New Orleans is rebuilding its ruined school system from the ground up. *Governing.* May 28, 2013. Available at: http://www.governing.com/blogs/bfc/col-rebuilding-new-orleans-public-schools.html. Accessed October 22, 2016.

45. Greening of New Orleans—10 years after Hurricane Katrina. *Green Money Journal.* October 2015. Available at: http://greenmoneyjournal.com/new-orleans. Accessed August 9, 2017.

46. Louisiana Recovery School District. New Orleans school facilities master plan. 2014. Available at: http://rsdla.net/apps/pages/index.jsp?uREC_ID=195282&type=d. Accessed October 22, 2016.

47. LEED for schools: Andrew H. Wilson Elementary School New Orleans. New Orleans, LA: HMS Architects; 2007.

48. Dreilinger D. InspireNOLA will take over Andrew Wilson Charter School in New Orleans. *The Times-Picayune.* March 14, 2016. Available at: http://www.nola.com/education/index.ssf/2015/02/inspirenola_will_take_over_and.html. Accessed October 22, 2016.

49. Morris R. Parents seethe over loss of charter at Wilson school in Broadmoor. *Uptown Messenger.* January 21, 2015. Available at: http://uptownmessenger.com/2015/01/parents-seethe-over-loss-of-charter-at-wilson-school-in-broadmoor. Accessed October 22, 2016.

11

KEEPING ABREAST OF ISSUES, MODELS, DATA SETS, AND TOOLS

Chapters 5 through 10 described and illustrated 18 tool sets that have proven to add value to public health and planning practice. However, new data sets, methods, models, and tools will follow in the wake of new challenges. This final chapter focuses on the Internet as the place to which we increasingly turn to keep abreast of issues and tools.

Before getting into details about specific Web sites, we begin by recognizing an undeniable trend toward so-called big data information systems. Practically speaking, this means open-source data from traditional phone surveys and government censuses, but also from Internet tools that will rapidly obtain, integrate, and publish data. Big data allows for the testing of methods and models that can clarify associations among variables and simulate alternative impacts if one of those variables is changed.

Journals

Notwithstanding this trend toward use of the Web, journals and books are the first place to look for new methods and information about new tools because the peer-review process, despite its warts, tends to recognize the most interesting ideas. Hence, we begin with an alphabetical list of the journals that we routinely check. In reality, this list could easily have exceeded 50.

- *American Journal of Preventive Medicine*
- *American Journal of Public Health*
- *Annual Review of Public Health*
- *Environment and Planning A*
- *Environmental Health Perspectives*
- *Environmental Impact Assessment Review*
- *Environmental Planning and Management*
- *Environmental Science and Technology*
- *Health Affairs*

- *Journal of Planning Education and Research*
- *Journal of the American Planning Association*
- *Morbidity and Mortality Weekly Report*
- *Natural Hazards Review*
- *Risk Analysis, an International Journal*

Rather than search every issue of these and other journals, an alternative is to set up a Google Alerts account. Simply open the Google browser and type in "alerts" to begin the registration process. This entails choosing key words and then periodically checking the account for recent publications across a broad spectrum of journals. We also suggest that every reader create a Google Scholar Alerts account.

Web Sites

As former journal editors, we realize that journals can take one to three years to diffuse information. To be current, we need to turn to colleagues, professional meetings, and Web sites. Before writing this chapter, we spoke with researchers and agency experts, explained the content of this book, and produced the following alphabetical list of broad search terms that are related to public health and planning.

- Air quality or pollution
- Databases
- Economic development
- Environmental impact
- Environmental justice
- Food security
- Hazards
- Health impacts
- Healthy cities
- Healthy communities
- Healthy people
- Land use
- Models
- Public health
- Resilience
- Sustainability
- Tools/methods
- Urban planning
- Waste
- Water

One strategy for finding up-to-date information online is to search through specific Web sites, particularly ones that are well maintained. The five Web sites discussed in the following paragraphs have a similar style—that is, they have an A-to-Z search engine, present an organized history of various issues, and cover news and other highlights in their field. Following the descriptions of our five favorite Web sites, we include brief notes about 10 others.

The U.S. Environmental Protection Agency: https://www.epa.gov

All you need to type into a search engine is "epa.gov" and you will open a treasure trove of information. In fact, we consult this Web site about health and environmental issues more than any other one. The home page takes you to news releases and news; the U.S. Environmental Protection Agency's (EPA's) history, laws, and regulation; and the agency's A-to-Z search engine.

The EPA Web site's strength is also its weakness, a statement that is true of the majority of sites in this section. Because it provides a massive amount of information, finding exactly what you are looking for can be a challenge. For example, we have been keeping abreast and have written about the Flint, Michigan, water contamination case.[1] If you went to the A-to-Z index when this chapter was written, "Flint" was not listed under the "popular topics" on the home page. If you searched under "F" in the alphabetized set of references on the home page, you were directed to the "Flint Drinking Water Response." Although it is a report on Flint, it was not what we were looking for. What we wanted to know was whether or not the federal government has agreed to continue to provide water and other needed resources to Flint until the problem is remediated.

Our next attempt to find what we wanted sent us back to the A-to-Z search engine where we typed in "Flint, Michigan." This yielded more than 5,000 EPA reports and notes about Flint, not all of which were about the water quality issue. After four additional word combinations, we found what we were looking for: an August 3, 2016, news release that documents a federal government pledge to continue to support Flint for the foreseeable future, even though the State of Michigan will assume responsibility for paying for water as needed.[2] This search took more than 15 minutes.

Some issues, typically those that have a long-standing record with the EPA, are easier to find. For example, the Vineland Chemical Company in Vineland, New Jersey, manufactured herbicides until the late 1980s. These herbicides contained arsenic, resulting in serious land and water contamination on its 54-acre site and creating significant human health risk from ingestion of surface water, sediments, and biota in the area. We wanted to know how the cleanup of this Superfund site was progressing. It took 30 seconds to find the information we wanted, which was a scheduled meeting to consider EPA's proposals for the next steps in the cleanup. The information was at the top of a list of 854 entries about the Vineland site.[3] The historical organization of the entries about the site allowed the user to find important information in chronological order.

One slow day in the summer of 2016, we decided to measure the number of citations for 20 commonly used search terms on the EPA Web site. An enormous amount of information turned up, as shown by the number of citations in parentheses:

- Air quality (n=11,600)
- Databases (n=29,900)
- Economic development (n=8,900)
- Environmental impact (n=18,200)
- Environmental justice (n=9,850)
- Food security (n=26,200)
- Hazards (n=12,600)
- Health impacts (n=14,600)
- Healthy cities (n=39,400)
- Healthy communities (n=42,400)
- Healthy people (n=20,400)
- Land use (n=14,800)
- Public health (n=19,800)
- Models (n=18,800)
- Resilience (n=4,790)
- Sustainability (n=10,400)
- Tools/methods (n=8,390)
- Urban planning (n=14,800)
- Waste (n=25,600)
- Water (n=39,100)

Many of the references only briefly mentioned the topic we were searching for, but it could take a long time to sort that out. One strategy to narrow the field of what you are looking for is to add an additional search term or date. For example, when we typed in "water, 2016," the number of references dropped from more than 39,000 to 5,030. When we added "news releases," it dropped to 2,270. EPA also allows the user to search under the categories of "environmental professionals" and "regulatory." When added to the search term "water," the number of citations was reduced even further.

Many users are only interested in their local area, so another way to narrow your search is by EPA region. Overall, searching by date, by EPA region, and for the most recent releases will reduce the number of citations for review. The more precise you can be, the more likely you will quickly find exactly what you are searching for. The problem with adding too many search terms, however, is that you may eliminate references that you really should review. Indeed, we admit that some of the more interesting information we have found while searching the EPA site was when we were actually searching for something else. On the other hand, we are happy to say that the days of sitting in the library looking for a few key citations are over.

EPA staff members are well aware of the complexity of their site. To help users, the agency produced targeted searches for methods, tools, models, and useful databases. For example, if you type in "methods, models, tools, and databases," you will be led to the Web page "Health Research Methods, Models, Tools, and Databases."[4] Multiple links are provided on this Web page so the user can connect to them for air, climate change, ecosystems, health, homeland security, human health risk assessment, land and waste management, safer chemicals, sustainable development, and water.

By scanning these links and others, the authors found three tools that have proven to be useful. In Chapter 7, we described and illustrated EJSCREEN, which is easy to use and allows the user to compare exposure and potential exposures in different areas.[5] MyEnvironment is a related second tool.[6] Type in the term and you will be guided to a tool that allows you to view EPA-collected information for neighborhoods on a map. You can enter your five-digit zip code, and the tool will produce a map, data, and graphics identifying the following kinds of data:

- Emergency incidents
- Superfund sites (CERCLA) and brownfields
- Toxic releases to the air and water (Toxic Release Inventory data; 8-hour ozone and fine particulate standards)
- Direct emissions into rivers, including toxic releases
- Cancer-causing agents in the area
- EPA water monitors and U.S. Geological Survey real-time water gauging stations

We put in the zip code of the area where our offices are located and found that it (1) violates the 8-hour ozone standard and (2) has a nontrivial amount of fine particulate matter (PM 2.5). The ozone standard is typically violated during the summer months along the entire Northeast corridor between Boston, Massachusetts, and Washington, D.C., as automobile engine emissions drift hundreds of miles eastward across the nation. Even rural areas in this corridor violate the ozone standard.

It is important to point out that the data available in these two toolkits should not be taken at face value. You may have hazardous waste sites, brownfields, factories, and other hazard substance emitters in a search area, but their presence does not imply that residents of that area are exposed. In fact, residents in your search area may be exposed to the same background level of exposure as are those in neighboring regions, or even less. Unfortunately, our experience has demonstrated that users tend to skip over the warnings about data limitations in these toolkits and go directly to making maps. While making maps may be fun, the results obtained from both EJSCREEN and MyEnvironment need careful vetting. Each tool takes about 45 minutes to understand, including reading about their limitations. We cannot overstate the limitations of the information produced from toolkits. On the other hand, our students enjoy using these in tools in our classes, particularly because they can compare different areas. We are careful to have them delve into the limitations sections before making in-class presentations so they can be good consumers of the information. We recommend that you do the same before presenting results from these toolkits at public meetings.

EPA's Community-Focused Exposure Risk and Sustainability Tool (C-FERST)[4,7] is an ambitious effort to establish a database with accompanying models that illustrate the big data approach for public health and planning at the local scale. C-FERST is an online tool that allows communities to access EPA data sets, fact sheets about chemicals, and mapping tools to enable community groups to gain a better understanding of the measurable threats to human health and safety in their neighborhoods. The tool includes links to what EPA identifies as sustainable management ideas. In essence, the tool allows local stakeholders and EPA officials to conduct their own exposure assessments of small areas. The essence of the tool is as follows:

- Maps of community environmental information, including demographics, pollution sources, and estimated concentrations and exposures.
- Comparison of these results with county and state estimates, which provides stakeholders with a local and statewide perspective on their own environment.
- Access to profiles created elsewhere that add further context about conditions and other environments.
- Hotlinks that allow the community to read what other areas have done in regard to exposure and risk reduction management options.
- Assistance with providing a local environmental health assessment.

The reader will recognize that the first two of these five are the essence of the EJSCREEN and MyEnvironment tools. Zartarian and colleagues[8] assert that C-FERST is the "flagship tool" for cumulative exposure assessment developed by EPA's National Exposure Laboratory.

C-FERST has been piloted in communities, typically communities with environmental justice challenges, that EPA has been working with. We assess it to be at the early stages, and so it is not reasonable to conclude how valuable it will be to readers of this book. It is not difficult, however, to envision more data, more models, and more opportunities to use this approach for building local consensus around risk management priorities. It could be an excellent example of an open-source and widely used data tool that increases community involvement and builds trust. For example, we can envision noise, odors, and other issues being added to the database, and we fully expect nonchemical agents to be included. On the other hand, it is also possible that the early tests of this tool will not go well and that ongoing opposition to EPA's environmental justice program by some elected officials will lead to cancellation or limited funding of this and similar efforts.

Centers for Disease Control and Prevention: https://www.cdc.gov

Along with the EPA site, the Centers for Disease Control and Prevention's (CDC's) is the Web site we most frequently search. It has many of the same assets as the EPA one. For example, there is a news section, a message from the CDC director, discussions about CDC's science programs, and its history. The user can access *The Morbidity and Mortality Weekly Report*[9] (*MMWR*), which summarizes key public health studies and news, particularly about disease outbreaks. Given CDC's central role across the breadth of public health issues, readers will find a great deal about health care on the Web site. For example, health care costs are high, and estimating those costs is important to states. Hence, CDC developed a chronic disease cost calculator for state governments to use.[10] The tool provides state-level estimates of medical expenditures and absenteeism costs for arthritis, asthma, cancer, cardiovascular diseases, depression, and diabetes.

Like the EPA site, it can sometimes be hard to find exactly what you want, but then there is much to find that relates to both planning and public health. We entered "toolkit" into the search box and came up with many pages of listings. Most of the listings were dedicated to individual diseases or information for health care workers, but some were particularly useful for both planners and public health practitioners. For example, the Healthy Places[11] Web site explains that, in 2002, the American Planning Association adopted a definition of Smart Growth (see Chapter 2) that seeks to create communities for all that

- Have a unique sense of community and place.
- Preserve and enhance valuable natural and cultural resources.
- Equitably distribute the costs and benefits of development.
- Expand the range of transportation, employment, and housing choices in a fiscally responsible manner.
- Value long-range, region-wide sustainability rather than short-term, incremental, or geographically isolated actions.
- Promote public health and healthy communities.

Contemporaneously with the emergence of Smart Growth, CDC launched a Built Environment and Health Initiative to improve public health through healthy community design by

- Increasing physical activity.
- Reducing injury.
- Increasing access to healthy food.
- Improving air and water quality.
- Minimizing the effects of climate change.

- Decreasing mental health stresses.
- Strengthening the social fabric of the community.
- Providing fair access to livelihood, education, and resources.

To achieve these objectives, the agency provides links to several tools and toolkits on its Web site. For example, there is a Healthy Community Design Checklist Tool,[12] a How-to Guide for Creating a Health Profile of Your Neighborhood,[13] a Health Communicator's Social Media Toolkit,[14] a Built Environment (BE) Assessment Tool,[15] and a Transportation Health Impact Tool,[16] among others. There is also a separate Web page that links to tools for creating health impact assessments.[17] (See Chapter 5 for further information on checklists and health impact assessments.)

We found the BE tool quite interesting.[15] It aids the user in measuring core features of their community, particularly

- BE infrastructure (road types, curb cuts and ramps, intersections and crosswalks, traffic control, and public transportation)
- Walkability (safe, attractive sidewalks and paths with inviting features)
- Bikeability (bike lanes or bike path features)
- Recreational sites and structures (parks, ball fields, and amenity features)
- Food environment (grocery stores, convenience stores, food kiosks, and farmers markets)

As planners and public health professionals often have different professional vocabularies, the BE tool provides a platform for them to jointly understand how the built environment impacts community health. It also identifies areas where they can collaborate to make their community a healthier place.

As with the toolkits listed under the EPA Web site, the CDC toolkits come with an explanation that the data have limitations. Users are encouraged to read these limitations carefully before coming to conclusions about the results. This also applies to the toolkits provided by the CDC's groups. We recommend that you search for tools provided by the three groups listed in Table 11.1.

We searched the Agency for Toxic Substances and Disease Registry (ATSDR) Web site and found both the ATSDR Communications Toolkit[19] and a Community Concern Assessment Tool.[21] The Community Concern Assessment Tool uses an 11-question survey to determine whether the level of concern about a health-related issue in a community is "high concern, high risk," "high concern, low risk," or "low concern, high risk." After assessing the level of concern, the tool then provides recommendations for how to communicate with the community about that risk. For example, let us suppose that there is high concern about a local toxic spill, but low risk except to those who might have direct contact with the agent. What tone and strategies should you use to address the concerns of the community? The tool makes suggestions for how to appropriately and effectively communicate with the public for each concern or risk scenario.

Table 11.1. Selected Centers for Disease Control and Prevention Groups and Associated Sites

CDC Group	Web Site	Comments
Agency for Toxic Substances and Disease Registry (ATSDR)	http://www.atsdr.cdc.gov	This site contains a long list of potentially valuable information, including disease registries, toxicological profiles, fact sheets, case studies, and brownfield redevelopment. The Web site has a link to a tool: ATSDR Brownfield and Land Reuse Site Tool.[18]
National Center for Environmental Health	https://www.cdc.gov/nceh	This site contains links to valuable health and environmental data resources, as well as multiple environmental health toolkits and social media tools. It links to an important tool: ATSDR Communication Toolkit.[19]
Office of Disease Prevention and Health Promotion	https://health.gov https://www.healthypeople.gov https://healthfinder.gov	These sites contain news, reports, and links to tools and data sets related to *Healthy People 2020* objectives, which include many issues discussed in this book. Of note is the link to Public Health 3.0,[20] which recognizes that the environment is a more important determinant of health than an individual's genetic code.

Note: CDC = Centers for Disease Control and Prevention.

Federal Emergency Management Agency: https://www.fema.gov

Given the markedly increased environmental devastation and costs associated with natural hazard events, the Federal Emergency Management Agency's (FEMA's) Web site is a must for local and state-level practitioners. Organizationally located within the U.S. Department of Homeland Security, FEMA's charge is to support first responders and the public in preparing, protecting against, responding to, and recovering from hazard events. Hazard mitigation plans are probably the most obvious manifestation of that responsibility, but not the only one. Table 11.2 summarizes areas of FEMA responsibilities with search terms to the various Web sites and tools.

National Association of County and City Health Officials: http://naccho.org

The National Association of County and City Health Officials (NACCHO) is a not-for-profit association serving about 3,000 local, regional, state, and tribal health departments in the United States from a home office in Washington, D.C. Along with an A-to-Z search engine, NACCHO'S pragmatic orientation is marked by the NACCHO toolbox and alerts accessed through Twitter (http://twitter.com/NACCHOalerts).

Table 11.2. Selected FEMA Agency Web Resources: https://www.fema.gov

Group Focus	Enter Into Search Box	Comments
Climate change	climate-change	Good way of keeping track of FEMA's climate-focused work with other government and private organizations.
Economic impact of hazard events	hazus	Tool used in natural hazard economic impact studies. Users' group can be helpful in noting limitations and providing assistance.
Flood insurance	national-flood-insurance-program	Critical program that advises local governments on how to reduce costs and participate in government-sponsored programs.
Flood mapping	national-flood-insurance-program/flood-hazard-mapping	Provides assistance on how to use and keep abreast of local flood hazard maps.
Hazard mitigation planning	hazard-mitigation-planning	Keeping up to date with this evolving national program is essential.
Historic preservation	office-of-environmental-planning-and-historic-preservation	Ideas about preserving local historical and cultural assets.

Note: FEMA = Federal Emergency Management Agency.

NACCHO has a broad agenda that can be conveniently divided into the following four areas:

- Community health, including adolescent, child, and maternal health; chronic disease and infectious disease prevention; immunization; injury reduction; and health equity.
- Public health infrastructure, which means improving the quality of public health services and measuring their quality.
- Public health preparedness, which has focused on preparedness for disease outbreaks, including assembling strategic stockpiles.
- Environmental health, including a broad set of interconnected topics, such as environmental justice, climate change, food safety, and environmental assessment.

In essence, NACCHO is a liaison between the federal government and local health departments. It provides training courses and meetings, access to information that can be used by local health departments in campaigns, and grants to increase preparedness and food security, including tools that are developed by NACCHO and/or by individual departments. Also, NACCHO is a key player advocating in Congress for improving public health in the United States. In short, NACCHO is a leader, a provocateur, and a catalyst for local governments.

One need not be a local health official to have access to NACCHO's Web site. We strongly suggest that you review NACCHO's toolbox, which is online and provides a free set of tools for local public health. These consist of fact sheets, full presentations, protocols, drills, evaluations, templates, and other types of tools. As of 2016, more than 130 of these tools were accessible. Some of our favorites focus on the following:

- Access to public rights-of-way
- Brownfields
- Health equity
- Health impact assessment
- Land use
- Promoting active living communities
- Transportation

Some of these tools were originally developed by local health departments; others were developed with federal agencies such as EPA and CDC. The first author used an early and still useful walkability tool developed by the University of Delaware in a class with mostly freshmen and sophomores.[22] The tool explains its purpose, how to use it, and how to place it in the context of the larger municipality. The first nine questions rate walking assets on a 6-point scale (1 = excellent; 2 = very good; 3 = good; 4 = some problems; 5 = many problems; and 6 = awful). Individual questions then focus on access, safety, width, continuity, curb, cracks and breaks, and obstructions. The tool then zeroes in on what can be done, including the need for better signals, striped crosswalks, ramps, benches, trees, lights, maintenance, and so on. Our students at first were not sure about why I wanted them to do this exercise. After they completed it, they admitted to enjoying it and felt as if it should be done for parts of their home communities.

The number of NACCHO tools will continue to expand; hence, the Web site should be a priority for searches relating to both public health and planning.

World Health Organization: http://www.who.int/en

The World Health Organization (WHO) manages international health programs for the United Nations. Because of its high credibility, WHO reports and suggestions are taken seriously by the overwhelming majority of nations and people. For example, WHO's International Agency for Research on Cancer (IARC) is assumed to be the leading expert on whether a substance is a carcinogen, a tumor promoter, or not a carcinogen. In June 2016, IARC declared that coffee is not a cause of bladder cancer and in fact has potential health benefits. It added that it might be hot beverages that increase the risk of bladder cancer. Individual researchers had also reached this conclusion, but it was not coincidental that two of our friends who had stopped drinking coffee years ago began drinking it again within a week of the IARC news release.

In addition to updates on carcinogens, WHO is the best site for staying abreast of worldwide efforts and updates about global health problems and efforts in the following areas:

- Environmental cancer
- Health impact assessment
- Health-related news from many countries
- Infographics (high-quality visual representations about epidemic disease threats, suicides, dementia, yellow fever, and other health-related issues—recommended for public discussions)
- Publications across a wide range of public health topics, ranging from psoriasis to outdoor air pollution
- Tools for both education and research

The WHO's portfolio is enormous. A search for toolkits yielded more than 3,700 links. We found, for example, a Recovery Toolkit for re-instituting health services after disasters.[23] We also found a toolkit for assessing human health risks from chemical exposures.[24]

As more toolkits are continuously being added, we recommend reviewing this resource for toolkits at least annually. WHO also provides data sets and reports on global health issues. The data sets include various health indicators and can be downloaded through GapMinder[25] or the Global Health Observatory.[26]

Briefer Treatment

Table 11.3 lists selected other organizations and their Web sites.

Final Thoughts

We have gone from a world where finding information required searching card catalogues and printed indexes (hoping the library had what we needed) to being able to find masses of potentially useful information without leaving our desks. The only downside is that it means sorting through enormous numbers of resources in a systematic manner so we can be kept abreast of current issues, ideas, tools, models, and data sets in our fields. The authors hope they have made the case that planning and public health are synergistic fields rather than professional silos. We also hope we have provided clear explanations of the tools and data sets listed in this book, demonstrated their usefulness with interesting case studies, and provided public health and planning professionals with useful links that will aid them in jointly making their communities healthier places to live.

Table 11.3. Other Recommended Web Sites

Group	Web Site	Comments
American Planning Association (APA)	https://www.planning.org	APA provides education for planning professionals, including the leading planning journal (*JAPA*). It has a Facebook page and provides Web tools, as well as books that contain valuable information on topics discussed in this book (see also Chapter 2).
American Public Health Association (APHA)	https://www.apha.org http://ajph.aphapublications.org http://thenationshealth.aphapublications.org	APHA publishes the leading public health professional journal (*AJPH*), books, and a society newspaper, (*Nation's Health*), and has a Facebook page and other Web site tools (see also Chapter 3).
Congress for the New Urbanism (CNU)	https://www.cnu.org	CNU provides design ideas, reports, and other information about the use of design to create healthier environments (see also Chapter 2).
National Hazards Center at the University of Colorado (NHC)	https://hazards.colorado.edu	NHC has a long history of commenting on key issues and providing extensive citations to the black and gray literatures about natural hazards.
Natural Resources Defense Council (NRDC)	https://www.nrdc.org	NRDC provides comments and policy suggestions about key environmental, health, and land use issues, such as climate change, communities, energy, food, oceans, and water, among others.
U.S. Census Bureau	https://www.census.gov	The Census Bureau provides data and tools essential to planning and public health practice.
U.S. Department of Agriculture (USDA)	https://www.usda.gov	USDA is deeply involved in measuring land use changes, posthazard events on the ground impacts, and climate change impacts.
U.S. Department of Energy (DOE)	https://energy.gov	The energy science and nuclear waste management groups within DOE have their own Web sites that focus on multiple key issues for planning and public health.
U.S. Department of the Interior (DOI)	https://www.doi.gov	DOI has major missions that include natural and cultural resources management.
U.S. Department of Transportation (DOT)	https://www.transportation.gov	DOT has valuable survey tools, data, and models that can be applied to a wide variety of applications.

References

1. Greenberg MR. Delivering fresh water: critical infrastructure, environmental justice, and Flint, Michigan. *Am J Public Health*. 2016;106(8):1358–1360.

2. US Environmental Protection Agency. Officials emphasize commitment to Flint after federal emergency declaration expires. August 11, 2016. Available at: https://www.epa.gov/newsreleases/officials-emphasize-commitment-flint-after-federal-emergency-declaration-expires. Accessed September 2, 2016.

3. US Environmental Protection Agency. EPA proposes expanded cleanup for old pesticide plant in Vineland, NJ. July 22, 2016. Available at: https://www.epa.gov/newsreleases/epa-proposes-expanded-cleanup-old-pesticide-plant-vineland-nj. Accessed September 2, 2016.

4. US Environmental Protection Agency. Methods, models, tools, and databases. 2016. Available at: https://www.epa.gov/research/methods-models-tools-and-databases. Accessed September 2, 2016.

5. US Environmental Protection Agency. EJSCREEN: Environmental Justice Screening and Mapping Tool. 2016. Available at: https://www.epa.gov/ejscreen. Accessed March 14, 2017.

6. US Environmental Protection Agency. MyEnvironment. Envirofacts. 2016. Available at: https://www3.epa.gov/enviro/myenviro. Accessed September 2, 2016.

7. US Environmental Protection Agency. Community-Focused Exposure and Risk Screening Tool (C-FERST). 2016. Available at: https://www.epa.gov/healthresearch/community-focused-exposure-and-risk-screening-tool-c-ferst. Accessed September 2, 2016.

8. Zartarian VG, Schultz BD, Barzyk TM, et al. The Environmental Protection Agency's Community-Focused Exposure and Risk Screening Tool (C-FERST) and its potential use for environmental justice efforts. *Am J Public Health*. 2011;101(suppl 1):S286–S294.

9. Centers for Disease Control and Prevention. *Morbidity and Mortality Weekly Report (MMWR)*. Available at: http://www.cdc.gov/mmwr/index.html. Accessed September 2, 2016.

10. Centers for Disease Control and Prevention. Chronic disease cost calculator. 2015. Available at: http://www.cdc.gov/chronicdisease/calculator. Accessed September 2, 2016.

11. Centers for Disease Control and Prevention. Healthy Places. 2014. Available at: https://www.cdc.gov/healthyplaces/about.htm. Accessed March 14, 2017.

12. Centers for Disease Control and Prevention. Healthy Community Design Checklist Toolkit. 2013. Available at: http://www.cdc.gov/healthyplaces/toolkit. Accessed March 14, 2017.

13. Centers for Disease Control and Prevention. Creating a health profile of your neighborhood: a how-to-guide. Available at: https://www.cdc.gov/healthyplaces/toolkit/sources_of_health_data.pdf. Accessed September 3, 2016.

14. Centers for Disease Control and Prevention. The Health Communicator's Social Media Toolkit. 2011. Available at: http://www.cdc.gov/healthcommunication/toolstemplates/socialmediatoolkit_bm.pdf. Accessed September 3, 2016.

15. Centers for Disease Control and Prevention. The Built Environment Assessment Tool Manual. 2015. Available at: http://www.cdc.gov/nccdphp/dch/built-environment-assessment. Accessed March 14, 2017.

16. Centers for Disease Control and Prevention. Transportation and Health Tool. 2015. Available at: https://www.cdc.gov/healthyplaces/healthtopics/transportation/tool.htm. Accessed March 14, 2017.

17. Centers for Disease Control and Prevention. Health impact assessment. 2016. Available at: https://www.cdc.gov/healthyplaces/hia.htm. Accessed March 14, 2017.

18. Agency for Toxic Substances and Disease Registry. ATSDR Brownfield/Land Reuse Health Program: ATSDR Brownfields/Land Reuse Site Tool. 2014. Available at: http://www.atsdr.cdc.gov/sites/brownfields/site_inventory.html. Accessed July 19, 2017.

19. Agency for Toxic Substances and Disease Registry. ATSDR Communication Toolkit. 2015. Available at: http://www.atsdr.cdc.gov/communications-toolkit/c7.html. Accessed March 14, 2017.

20. Office of Disease Prevention and Health Promotion, Centers for Disease Control and Prevention. Public Health 3.0. 2016. Available at: https://www.healthypeople.gov/2020/tools-resources/public-health-3. Accessed March 14, 2017.

21. Agency for Toxic Substances and Disease Registry. Community Concern Assessment Tool. 2015. Available at: http://www.atsdr.cdc.gov/communications-toolkit/documents/08_community-concern-assessment-tool_508.pdf. Accessed September 3, 2016.

22. O'Hanlon J, Scott J. Healthy Communities: The Walkability Assessment Tool. Newark, DE: Institute for Public Administration, University of Delaware; 2010.

23. Recovery Toolkit: Supporting Countries to Achieve Health Service Resilience. Geneva, Switzerland: World Health Organization; 2016.

24. WHO Human Health Risk Assessment Toolkit: Chemical Hazards. Geneva, Switzerland: World Health Organization; 2010.

25. Gapminder. Data in Gapminder World. Available at: https://www.gapminder.org/data. Accessed March 14, 2017.

26. World Health Organization. Global Health Observatory data. 2016. Available at: http://www.who.int/gho/en. Accessed September 3, 2016.

INDEX